By His Stripes

The story of one woman's courageous fight of faith against cancer and miraculous healing through the living Word of God

By

Deborah M. West

*Cathey'
For His Glory
Deborah
1 Peter 2:24*

ISBN: 1-4140-3628-0 (e-book)
ISBN: 1-4140-3626-4 (Paperback)
ISBN: 1-4140-3627-2 (Dust Jacket)

Library of Congress Control Number: 2004090218

This book is printed on acid free paper.

Printed in the United States of America
Bloomington, IN

Scriptures taken from the *New King James Version*.

1stBooks - rev. 01/12/04

Disclaimer:

This book is not intended to provide medical advice or to take the place of medical advice and treatment from your personal physician. Readers are advised to consult their own doctors or other qualified health professionals regarding the treatment of their medical problems. Neither the publisher nor the author takes any responsibility for any possible consequences from any action or application of medicine, supplement, herb or preparation by any person reading or following the information in this book.

Acknowledgments

"Walking with Deborah and Charlie through their trial with cancer was something to behold. Watching their faith and determined obedience to find God's will in harmony with God's Word was a powerful experience. This book tells that story in a compelling and fascinating way."

L. H. Hardwick, Jr. ,Senior Pastor
Christ Church, Nashville, Tennessee

"Deborah tackles the doubters of God's healing in a straightforward style. Through scripture and her own journey, she lays out the truth of how God's Word is powerful and still applies in this day and age."

- Dave Ramsey, *New York Times* Best Selling Author and National Radio Talk Show Host of *'The Dave Ramsey Show'*

"A truly inspiring story of courage and faith in the face of a devastating diagnosis — may all who read *By His Stripes* realize that God is a very present help in time of trouble."

- Nancy Alcorn, President and founder of Mercy Ministries of America, and author of *Echoes of Mercy*.

Dedication

This book is dedicated to my loving husband, Charlie, who stood with me steadfast in faith, knowing that God is not a man that He should lie; His Word is truth.

One can chase a thousand, but two can put ten thousand to flight (Deuteronomy 32:30). And to God, for the dedication of His Son, by whose stripes I am healed.

"But indeed for this purpose I have raised you up, that I may show My power in you, and that My name may be declared in all the earth," (Exodus 9:16).

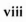

Table of Contents

Foreword

I will never forget the day Deborah West told me that she had been diagnosed with breast cancer. I remember so many things racing through my mind…*Why Deborah? She doesn't deserve this, she is so nice to everyone and she does so much for God. This is not fair! How would I feel if this were me?* The thoughts went on and on.

Deborah and her husband, Charlie, had become very strong supporters of Mercy Ministries. They were continuously volunteering their catering services as well as providing financial support to help us in reaching out to troubled young girls with the love of Christ. It was just a couple of weeks before that they had been over to cater an open house for our Nashville area supporters. This wonderful couple, so vibrant and full of life—how could tragedy strike so suddenly?

It is one thing to know "in principle" that we are healed by the stripes of Jesus, yet it is another thing altogether to know that your very life depends upon the manifestation of this truth in your physical body.

By His Stripes is a true story about a *real* woman who faced a *very real problem*—one that many thought would end her life. No matter what problem you or someone you love might be facing, you are sure to be inspired by this courageous woman who dared to confront the "facts" of her devastating diagnosis with the *truth* of God's Word.

I am so proud of Deborah for sharing with others her personal journey about how she experienced death being swallowed up in victory. May all who read this powerful story realize that God is a very present help in time of trouble (Psalm 46:1).

Nancy Alcorn
President and Founder
Mercy Ministries of America

Chapter 1

My Journey Begins

My journey is one of great tragedy, great trial, and great triumph. I want to take you down the road I traveled—through the cancer, past the fear and the bad reports—all the way through to the victory God promised me, and that I know awaits you. It is a road of possibilities, for with God *all things* are possible! Won't you take a step and walk on the water with me? With the Word of God paving your path and the Holy Spirit guiding your steps, you will make it to the other side!

And so it began, early in the summer of 1995. I remember it as if it were yesterday. I discovered a lump in my right breast. My husband, Charlie, and I were preparing for bed, and as I lay down, my hand rested across my chest. There it was: a lump the size and consistency of a pencil eraser. It was positioned near my breastbone, away from the dense, breast tissue.

A million and one thoughts flooded my mind, but reason quickly replaced question as I recalled statistics I had learned about this sort of thing. I had, after all, some history of cysts. I was sure this tiny lump was nothing.

Charlie's presence as he climbed into bed beside me jolted my thoughts to a halt long enough for me to disclose my curious finding. Charlie nodded a confirming yes; he saw it too. "It's probably a good idea to have the doctor check it out," he suggested. Sensing no cause for alarm, we did little more than agree upon my seeing the doctor before we drifted off to sleep.

I was reminded of the lump the next morning as I showered and dressed for the day. *I suppose a visit to the doctor wouldn't hurt,* I reasoned. After breakfast, I thumbed through my address book and located Dr. Presley's number. He was my long-time OBGYN and a man I highly respected as a healthcare professional. I phoned his office and described to his nurse the lump I had found the previous evening. She definitely thought I should have the doctor take a look at it, so she fit me into the schedule for later in the week.

Dr. Presley sounded concerned, but not alarmed, as he spoke to me after the exam. He instructed me to schedule a mammogram as soon as possible. I intended to do so, but thought I would wait until things slowed down at work before making the appointment. Charlie and I had established a successful catering business, and at times worked around the clock to meet the needs of our customers. *I'll just push this appointment out to a more convenient time*, I thought. However, that time would not come for quite a while.

Tragedy Hits Home

Within the next weeks came a devastating blow: my Daddy was diagnosed with esophageal cancer. "No, not my Daddy," came my response of disbelief. "How could this be happening to *my* family?" I questioned.

Somehow, in the blur of events to follow, I never scheduled the mammogram. Between caring for Daddy and working, my needs fell through the cracks. Life as we knew it was turned upside down and inside out, and what once seemed so important in our own day-to-day routine became insignificant in the face of this weightier, more eternal matter. Anyone who has cared for someone in the final stages of life knows the intense demands such a situation brings. The task is all-consuming of your thoughts, your emotions, your physical strength, and your time. But gladly, we all did our part: Mother, Peggy, Louise, Gail, Charlie, and me. We did what we knew to do, which, unfortunately, wasn't enough.

Daddy died October 5, 1995, only three short months after having been diagnosed. His passing was so sudden, and I remember asking God, "Wasn't there more we could have done?" Somehow, deep in my heart, I knew the answer had to be yes. Surely, God's best for His precious children is not to be viciously robbed of health and life. We would have done anything to keep Daddy from suffering so, but we didn't know there was anything else to do other than what the doctors told us. Though I didn't see it until much later, Daddy's experience with cancer was really the beginning of my quest to know more about the nature of God as Father and Jesus as Healer.

The decisions that followed Daddy's death filled our days. Where would Mother live? What would we do with the house? Who would handle the mounting pile of paperwork? So much needed to be done, and on top of all these details, we were still grieving our significant loss. Eight months had flown by before I finally called Dr. Presley to schedule a follow up exam.

It was now February 13, 1996, and surprisingly, I hadn't thought much about the lump. It seemed there were more important things to occupy my mind than myself. Besides, I had been diagnosed at age twenty-seven with Fibrocystic "Disease", the most common cause of breast lumps in women ages thirty-five to fifty, and the cause of eighty percent of all breast operations performed. Studies show that this condition, which is not an actual disease, is most likely caused by the mammary glands', ducts', and fibrous tissues' reaction to abnormal hormone levels. As a result, multiple pockets of fluid called sacs or cysts develop and an increase in fibrous tissue may form. In some instances, a lump may consist only of fibrous, rubbery tissue, a condition called Mammary Dysplasia. Tenderness and lump size commonly increase during the week before menstruation and decrease a week after. Fibrocystic Disease usually disappears after menopause. (Krames Communications, Robert M. Kradjian, MD, Breast Surgery.)

Having this medical knowledge, I reasoned that for someone with my medical history, having a lump didn't seem all that serious.

Apparently, Dr. Presley wasn't as convinced. The morning after my second appointment, he called to tell me that he had scheduled me for a mammogram the next day at the Baptist Hospital's Women's Pavilion in Nashville. That didn't concern me. I respected Dr. Presley and was sure he was just taking every precaution he felt was necessary.

Interestingly enough, when I had the mammogram done, the lump went undetected. I suspect because of its placement. Not satisfied with the findings, however, the doctor sent me to have an ultrasound, which showed the lump very clearly.

Dr. Huff was the radiologist reading the ultrasound. He was a kind and gentle man. We exchanged pleasant conversation during my visit and then I returned home. As I did after every visit to the doctor, I gave Charlie a detailed progress report. We felt confident that everything was ticking along like clockwork. Not one of the doctors seemed overly concerned, though the tests and referrals persisted.

The next day, Dr. Presley called and told me I needed to make an appointment to see Dr. Albert Spaw, a surgeon at Baptist Hospital. *Oh no, a surgeon,* I thought. I knew what that meant: they wanted to remove the lump. I scheduled a time to see Dr. Spaw the afternoon of February 28. As I spoke with the doctor the day of my appointment, I learned that he was a Christian man, as were all of the doctors who practiced together in the OBGYN group.

"Why did they send you here?" Dr. Spaw asked me as he began his exam.

I explained that I had found a lump in my right breast, and that Dr. Presley wanted him to look at it. He sorted through the ultrasound pictures and proceeded to present me my options. He said we could do a needle aspiration right then while I was there in his office, or remove the lump in two to three months. I knew our work schedule coming up was hectic; in the catering business some of our busiest months are September through May, and waiting three months would put us right at the tail end of our heaviest season.

"It's whatever *you* want to do," Dr. Spaw consoled, sensing my hesitation.

I opted for a date sooner than later, and worked with the office staff to settle on March 11. However, another dilemma confronted us: Charlie and I had no health insurance. That ruled out having the surgery at Baptist Hospital, and warranted the procedure as outpatient at the Nashville Surgery Center due to cost.

'Everything will be Fine'

The morning of March 11 came. Charlie and I arrived at the Surgery Center at 5:30 A.M., filled out paperwork, and waited. At 6:30 A.M., my name was called and I was sent to be prepped for surgery. The room was so cold! I shivered under the thin, cotton gown and was so thankful they allowed me to wear socks! First, the anesthesiologist came to administer the anesthesia. He was kind and comforting, taking time to talk with me as the drugs took effect. Next, Dr. Spaw arrived. I must admit it was reassuring to see a familiar face. "This won't take long," came his convincing words. "By 10 o'clock you will be on your way home."

Sure enough, by 9:45 I was roused to consciousness, though I was still groggy. Dr. Spaw explained to Charlie and me that he removed a small tumor about the size of a lima bean. He said that it was nothing and that everything would be fine. Charlie and I breathed a sigh of relief. Ready to put the succession of appointments, doctors, and tests behind me, I rested confidently in those words: "It's nothing…everything will be fine."

On our way home from the Center, Charlie needed to stop and pick up some lunch items for a box lunch order we had the next day. Before we got to the store however, the effects of the anesthesia began to take a toll on my body. Dizzy and nauseated I was feeling sicker by the minute. We made it into the Sam's parking lot just in time for the little bit of food that was in me to come out. Charlie hurried in and out of the store and whisked me home to rest. Fortunately, that was the first and last experience of its kind. The entire recovery process was amazingly fast and seamless, and in a matter of days I was doing the things I loved to do.

For some, that's where the journey ends; but for me, it was only beginning. Ahead lay a long road of unknowns with perhaps the greatest challenge of my life waiting just around the corner. Little did I know that along with the difficulties to come, I would also encounter the strength of a friend who would take me by the hand and guide me faithfully every step of the way. Charlie and I were about to embark on a greater adventure with God and His Word than we could have ever imagined. What a road we were about to travel—a road of pure faith!

Chapter 2

When Adversity Comes

Signs of spring were determined to prevail against the chilly March wind, hinting that winter would soon be behind us. I have always loved this time of year. Everything is crisp and fresh, and the hope of new life budding is not far off. Somehow, I felt the season paralleled my own life, representing closure to the past and expectancy for a bright future.

My recovery was going so well that Charlie and I decided to go shopping that afternoon at a favorite spot, a fun, catchall store where one could find just about anything imaginable. The day was Wednesday, March 13, just two days after the surgery. We hadn't driven five minutes from the house when my pager went off. It was Dr. Spaw's office. I looked at Charlie, puzzled. *Whatever could Dr. Spaw want?* I wondered. *He said everything looked good.*

I dialed his office on the cell phone and waited: one, two, three rings. The moment I heard Dr. Spaw's voice on the receiving end I knew something was wrong.

His words pierced the still air and reverberated in my ears, "Deborah, you have breast cancer."

Stunned, I sat speechless for a moment, then managed a dumbfounded, "Well, now what do we do?"

The next step was to schedule a consultation with Dr. Spaw to discuss my prognosis and treatment. Mechanically, I spoke with his nurse to pencil in a time for the following week, March 19, at 11:30 A.M.

Hearing the doctor's grim report felt like being hit in the face with a cinder block; which, mind you, is much larger than a brick. I stared straight ahead as Charlie drove and tried to decipher the notes I had scratched on a piece of paper while talking with the doctor.

We drove on to the store, which usually gave us so much pleasure. Seldom did we visit without collecting all sorts of treasures for our catering business or home. But today was just not the same. The doctor's words had knocked the wind from our sails. Life-threatening news affects different people in different ways. As for Charlie and me, we seemed to have no words to speak. In retrospect, saying *nothing* was probably the best thing we could have done at such a critical time. We have since learned the importance and power of our words, especially in the face of adverse circumstances. We have also learned that our heart can say one thing and our head another. It is wisdom to feed our spirit—our heart—with the Word of God, and then line our mouth up with what our heart says.

I can identify with those who hear devastating news pertaining to their own life or the life of a loved one. If you don't know what the Word of God says, you truly feel hopeless against the impending situation. I know I did. Certainly at the time, neither Charlie nor I knew anything about the healing message in the Bible. Such teachings were not part of the previous denominations we had been associated with all our lives. We were not hearing that Jesus bore *all* sickness and disease and that He provided healing for us every time—if we would believe and receive His Word. Our pastor believed that God healed him and his son, but I never heard him say God heals *all*. Friends from our church who believed that healing is for all would eventually share the healing message with me.

Salvation was the mainstay in the churches we had attended, and rightfully so. Besides, we hadn't done anything when Daddy was diagnosed with esophageal cancer just eight months ago. The doctors told us the cancer was at stage four, and there was nothing anyone could do anyway, except make him comfortable. He was given thirty-two radiation treatments, which only made him sick every day. After seeing what Daddy went through, Charlie and I were convinced there were five stages of cancer, one, two, three, four and *dead!*

Though neither one of us would admit it at the time, vivid pictures of Daddy's condition haunted us. We remembered how he had lost forty pounds in six weeks, how he couldn't hold himself up, and how

Deborah M. West

Mother, my sisters, and I cared for him until the day he died. I didn't know any better than to let such pictures play in my head, only this time casting myself as the main character. The road ahead appeared to be one I am sure many before me have traveled—a path paved with fear, worry, and a tragic end. Charlie and I looked at each other and began to cry. This wasn't at all what we expected. How does one prepare for such news?

As we sat side by side in the car that day, tears streaming down our faces, vivid memories of a cancer victim still fresh in our minds, and a road of uncertainty before us, we had nowhere to go but to God. We took one another by the hand and prayed. Though I don't recall the words we spoke, I know that we opened a door of faith that day, giving God the opportunity to move on our behalf. What we were facing was so much bigger than us and we needed help—divine help. That moment marked a significant turning point not only in our day, but also in our lives. Each decision we make, no matter how small, determines the direction our life will take. Whatever direction we travel ultimately determines our life's destiny. God had a destiny for my life and at that time I hadn't come close to fulfilling it. I suppose even now, after His faithful hand has guided me along such a challenging road, there is still more for me to discover. I do know this: part of my destiny is sharing with you what God brought me through. If you are on a road of despair, accelerating to what seems like a dead end, look up!

There is hope for you!

There is a way through!

There is a way to overcome, victoriously, and His Name is Jesus Christ!

Jesus is the Word of God made flesh, and the Bible says His Name is above every name, even "the name" of cancer.

The word cancer elicits a whole host of feelings and fears for most people. Many know the throws of its chilling sound because they recall loved ones the deadly disease has claimed. Others have survived cancer's attack, but I'm quite certain, not without some battle scars.

Charlie and I were no different. But if anything good came out of hearing those words "Deborah, you have cancer," it was that they brought us to a place of decision—a crossroads with two paths before us—a path of death and a path of life. The moment we chose to trust God in the face of impossible circumstances is the moment we chose a path of life; a way contrary to the way many choose, though unknowingly, sadly. "There is a way that seemeth right unto a man, but the end thereof are the ways of death" (Proverbs 16:25). Charlie and I chose to embark on a quest for the truth. This was territory unchartered by us, but thank God, He had already gone before us and prepared the way.

When we returned home from the store that day, I called my sisters, Peggy and Louise, to tell them the news. I decided not to call my sister Gail at that time, because my Mother lived with her and I didn't want Mother to know about the cancer just yet. The loss of her husband was still too recent, and I didn't want to burden her with anything more.

The doorbell rang sounding my sisters' arrival. I swallowed hard and took a deep breath before opening the door. Not sure of what to say or how to react, their faces showed strained emotion. They tried to be strong and pretend that everything was just fine, but all the while they were fighting back the tears.

Not long after they left, our phone started ringing. Word had gotten out among our Christian friends at church about the prognosis. Everyone was talking about the "C" word, as cancer is often called. Well into the evening the calls kept coming. With every one, I found myself repeating the doctor's report over and over again. The Word of God teaches that "Faith comes by hearing, and hearing…." I soon discovered that fear comes the same way! The more I talked the worse I felt. The spirit of fear was so heavy on me that I could physically feel its strong grip. Fear has a way of feeding itself, too. I felt compelled to call one of my friends, Gail Whited, to get some answers to the questions bombarding my mind. Gail was an outpatient surgical nurse at Baptist Hospital; she worked with my surgeon, Dr. Spaw. She told me just what I *thought* I wanted to know—which only added to the fear already consuming me.

After talking to Gail I made my way to our bedroom, where Charlie was reading in the sitting area. "Honey," I told him, "I am just riddled with fear."

Charlie always had a way of handling things. I knew I could tell him anything and he would find some way to make it better. As he always did, Charlie knew just what to say. "Do you know what *you* need to do, Deborah? *You* need to get alone with God and pray for His peace."

I knew he was right. He wasn't brushing me off or being uncompassionate. He was speaking the truth to me in love. Charlie knew not even he could handle this one for me; this was something I needed to do myself. We can't always depend on others to learn things for us, and perhaps I had done that more than I realized. I knew my relationship with the Lord was a strong one, and that I could depend on Him to help me through the long road ahead. The gentle nudge from Charlie helped me to recognize that.

Again, I had come to a point of decision and it was time to take another step. I found a secluded place in the house to be alone with God, to kneel, and to pray. I said what I knew to say to the Lord. I told Him I didn't understand what was happening to me or why, but that I would trust Him completely to see me through. I told Him I didn't mean to be afraid, but I just didn't know how not to be. I asked Him for His help and for His peace to settle over me. My words weren't fancy—they were honest. We have to be real with God if we want Him to be real to us. I believe God knew just how I felt, and He was simply waiting for me to turn everything over to Him so He could begin to work in my situation and show Himself strong on my behalf.

A Divine Dream

That night as I slept, the Lord revealed to me in a dream not only what He *could* do, but what He *would* do. He showed me that healing was His plan for me! It seems so simple to us that God *can* heal, but do we really believe and know that He *will* heal when we need healing and ask Him to heal? Healing itself was not a new concept to me; however, experiencing divine healing personally, was. Sure, I had read about Jesus and the disciples healing people in the Bible. I even knew people who had been healed. But now that I had been diagnosed with cancer, faced with the possibility of suffering and death, healing took on a whole new meaning to me. I was basically a blank slate. Having never been taught the healing message, I didn't have much to bank on in the area of healing until the Lord gave me this dream.

When I awoke the next morning, however, my thoughts instantly fell into the groove my fears and emotions were wearing in my mind the previous night. I sat alone at the breakfast table letting the tears roll down my face as I dwelled on "poor me." I recall telling the Lord, "I am not ready to die. I have young grandchildren and a fairly recent marriage of only six years. I know there is something more that I could do for You."

Then, as Charlie came to join me in the kitchen, all at once the dream came flooding back to me. Drying my tears I said to him, "Charlie, come sit down and let me tell you about the dream God gave me last night."

I shared with him how my Mother and my sister Peggy were standing to the right of me when an evil man got right up in my face, grabbed my right wrist (which was significant because the cancer was in my right breast), and proceeded to tell me as he jerked my arm straight out, "I'm going to destroy you." He took an object that resembled a small, sharp rake, and plunged it into my right wrist. As I looked down at my wrist, all I could see was blood spurting from every hole. It was horrifying. I cried out for Jesus to help me, and when I mentioned His Name, the evil man withered to the ground. Philippians 2:10–11 came alive to me: "That at the name of Jesus every knee should bow, of things in heaven, and things in earth, and things under the earth; And that every tongue should confess that Jesus Christ is Lord, to the glory of God the Father."

His knees bowed all right; he began to melt away under the Name of Jesus and its authority. To my amazement, when I turned around to show my Mother and sister what the man had done to my wrist, there was nothing there except a clean, healed scar. Instantly, I understood that Jesus had healed me from the evil attack.

Nothing like this had ever happened to me before. I had often heard of God speaking to people through dreams, but I had never experienced anything like this personally. Instead of tears of self-pity, I was now crying tears of joy! For the first time since I heard the doctor's grim words, I felt hope.

Charlie and I knew that regardless of what lay ahead, the outcome for me was total healing. No, God didn't show us every twist and turn along the road we would travel on this journey, but He did let us know we wouldn't be traveling alone. He would never leave us nor forsake us. He would be with us every step of the way just as He had promised in His Word.

If Two of You Agree

Charlie and I continued to pray and seek God about our next steps. As we did, God showed us that we were to set ourselves in agreement with the promises in His Word pertaining to healing. The only problem was, we didn't know what those promises were. It felt like we were on a treasure hunt, and as we diligently searched, we found the precious truths God had hidden for us, tucked away in His Word. His truth was there all along, it simply needed to be mined in order for us to make it our own.

Again I say unto you, That if two of you shall agree on earth as touching any thing that they shall ask, it shall be done for them of my Father which is in heaven.

Matthew 18:19

Agreement is a powerful force, and one of the things God put in our heart was to have other Christians agree with us for the healing we believed God had promised me. We began by calling Christian friends and customers to ask them to stand with us. At this particular turn, we encountered a huge obstacle. One of our customers worked for a Christian publisher, so I didn't think twice about calling her for support. To my surprise when I shared my request for her agreement of faith, I was confronted with words of doubt and despair. "You know Deborah, God doesn't always heal. He healed me of breast cancer, but He doesn't always choose to heal everyone."

As I sat on the living room sofa listening to her words strike me as arrows, my spirit on the inside shouted, "Hang up, you don't need to hear that!" Very graciously, I excused myself off the phone. I found Charlie in the next room and told him, "Well, we can mark her off our list; she doesn't believe God heals everyone."

What the enemy meant to be a boulder in my path, I used as a stepping stone to ground me even more firmly in faith. I dug my heels in and refused to let doubt diminish the new truth planted in my heart. My friend's words spawned a series of questions I couldn't help but ask. What made her so special that God *chose* to heal her? What did she do that was so exceptional? How did she know God was going to heal her? Nine years ago about that same time she had undergone a mastectomy and God saw her through it all. She looked wonderful and was still walking cancer-free. Though I praise God for the victory she experienced, I still turned the question over and over in my mind: *Why did God choose to heal her and not others?*

In my study of the Scriptures, I found that when Jesus walked this Earth He never refused to heal anyone. When He entered Capernaum or another city He didn't say, "Okay, everyone line up. I'm going to go down the line and pick and choose whom I want to heal today."

God is no respecter of persons (Acts 10:34). The Bible says that when we seek God we will find Him, when we seek Him with all our heart (Deuteronomy 4:29). Seeking God with all our heart is the key. I needed healing and so I had to seek God by learning His Word on the subject of healing. Believe me, it wasn't easy. If it were easy, I suppose more people would travel the path Charlie and I had chosen.

Satan put all kinds of roadblocks in my path, and he will do the same to you. I found myself giving all sorts of excuses for why I couldn't do this and why I didn't have time for that. After all, didn't God realize I had to work, take care of our house, go to church, and by all means keep up my volunteer commitments? Thank God I had Christian friends who knew what it was going to take for me to receive healing, and they obeyed God by continuously insisting that I do nothing but saturate myself in His Word.

Don't be surprised by the reactions of well-meaning people when you ask them to agree with you for your healing. Not all, but the majority of people we asked to pray for us thought we were "way out there." We could hear the skepticism in their voices. We couldn't let that bother us though; they didn't need healing from a deadly disease, I did. Remember, it is *your* faith—what *you* believe—that matters most.

Tuesday morning, March 19, I had a consultation scheduled with doctor Spaw. I hadn't planned on telling my Mother about the diagnosis until after my appointment, but a few days prior to the consultation, my sister Louise called. "You might as well call Mother and tell her," Louise advised, "she knows something is wrong."

How did she know? I can only assume it was the Holy Spirit "showing her things to come" to prepare her perhaps. He is, after all, our Comforter. It had only been eight months since her husband of sixty-one years had died of this horrible disease. Since that time God had shown Charlie and me so much more than we had ever known about healing. If only we had known then what we knew now, surely we would have used our faith and believed God for Daddy. But at the time he was diagnosed we didn't know to use our faith for healing because we had never been taught to do such a thing.

The fault is no one's but our own. We had Bibles; we even read them. And, we went to church. But that was part of the problem; no one at church ever taught healing. Yes, at my church we prayed for healing, but if healing didn't come, then it just wasn't God's will to heal. "To be absent from the body is to be present with the Lord," they always said. That is easy for people to say when it isn't them or one of their loved ones needing healing. I remember a church friend telling me that very thing one day. "Deborah, if you're not healed it will be a glorious thing to go home and be with the Lord." I thought later I would have liked to have told him, "Well then let's give your wife this disease instead of me and see how you feel about it." Yes, I know it will be glorious to be present with the Lord, but I just didn't think *now* was the time to go.

21

The time had come to tell Mother that the same deadly disease that prematurely took her husband's life was also attacking her "baby girl." This was one of the hardest things I had ever had to do. Friday morning I phoned, and knew instantly that what Louise had told me was right; Mother already knew something was wrong. "Mother," I told her, "I have been diagnosed with breast cancer."

Instantly, her tears began to flow. It was as if I could see right through the telephone to her lovely, kind face—a face filled at the moment with both compassion and fear. I sensed the Holy Spirit giving me all the right words to comfort her—words I couldn't have shared just eight short months ago. "Now Mother, I know you need to cry, but that isn't going to help me at all. After you're finished crying, the only thing that will help me is for you to agree with me for my healing."

I explained to her that Christ not only died for our sins, the Bible says He died for our sicknesses and diseases too (Isaiah 53:4–5). I know those words came right from heaven, because at that time I didn't have the revelation that salvation entailed healing from every sickness and disease. Though I believe she was comforted by those words, her doubt remained for the obvious reason: *Why wasn't her husband healed?* This was a question Charlie and I would soon be able to answer as we immersed ourselves in the Word of God.

Chapter 3

Turning a Corner

The day of our consultation with Dr. Spaw finally arrived. Charlie and I sat in the doctor's office attentively listening as he read the diagnosis: Right breast mass: In-situ and invasive adenocarcinoma with lobular features, 10mm maximum diameter, involving margin of biopsy. Hormone receptor report at the request of Dr. Albert Spaw, estrogen and progesterone receptors are performed using ERICA and PRICA methodology. There is strong nuclear staining for estrogen receptors and progesterone receptors in both the in-situ and invasive components. (John B. Thomison, Jr. M.D. SSM 031396.)

Dr. Spaw broke things down in layman's terms for us, and then explained the optional procedures. I had two choices: a mastectomy or a lumpectomy. He felt that a radical operation would not be necessary. His professional opinion was to perform a lumpectomy, which would involve removing the breast tissue that surrounded the initial lump. According to the Krames Communication publication entitled: *Breast Lumps – A Guide to Understanding Breast Problems and Breast Surgery,* a lumpectomy is often done in conjunction with an axillary dissection, the removal usually through a separate incision of some or most of the axillary (underarm) lymph nodes. Axillary dissection is often used both for treatment and to learn the possible extent of tumor growth. Axillary lymph nodes are small, bean-shaped glands that are linked in chains and extend up into the armpit. Lymph nodes act as lines of defense or filters against the spread of infection, much like that of a filter in an air conditioning or heating unit.

Dr. Spaw continued to explain that these "feelers", similar to the roots of a tree, remained after the tumor was removed. The biopsy revealed that the cancer cells were present all around the tumor's edges. He believed that if he went back in and removed more breast tissue as well as the lymph nodes, that he would remove all the cancer. However, if we chose the lumpectomy route, radiation therapy treatments would be necessary following the surgery. This procedure certainly sounded better than having my entire breast removed, so I opted for the lumpectomy.

As Charlie and I sat in Dr. Spaw's office, calmness settled over us. I knew we didn't have insurance, and I was sure the surgery and radiation treatments would be terribly expensive. Yet another opportunity for God to move! I made my way to the office manager's desk to discuss how I was going to pay for all of this, and to schedule future appointments. From where I stood, I remember peering through a little cubbyhole to where Dr. Spaw was typing at the computer inputting data. I glanced out the office window and was surprised to see a blanket of white; it was snowing like crazy. "I can't believe it's snowing" I commented, "it's almost the first day of spring and Friday is my birthday."

By the look on Dr. Spaw's face, it was if I had shot him right through the heart. "Oh Deborah, I wish I could have given you a better birthday present," he sighed as he made his way over to where I was standing. As he held out his arms to offer a consoling hug, I told him firmly, "Dr. Spaw, God can use you to heal me, or He can heal me on His own without you."

Surprised, he looked me right in the eyes and asked, "You have a lot of faith, don't you, Deborah?"

I guess I had never thought of my bold stand for healing as "faith." But indeed that is what it was. Truthfully, my response to Dr. Spaw's sympathetic tone surprised even me. I had always believed God for things, for jobs, for houses in which to live, and for my children, but now I was going to have to believe God for my life. That is truly the only fight we have been given; the good fight of faith (1 Timothy 6:12).

Whose Report Will You Believe?

Charlie and I had gone to church the Sunday night before my consultation. We had been attending Christ Church pastored by L. H. Hardwick for almost five years. We had grown strong in the Lord

25

there and had a wonderful network of friends. That night as we arrived, one of my friends, Gail Litteral, asked me, "Have you asked Pastor Stan to pray over you for healing?" Pastor Stan is an assistant pastor at Christ Church.

I told her I hadn't.

"We need to go and tell him right now," she insisted.

So, Gail and I took Pastor Stan aside and I shared the doctor's report with him. Of course it wasn't the report that Charlie and I believed; we were standing on the Word of God that says we are to believe the report of the Lord (Isaiah 53:1). Faith doesn't deny the facts, but in the face of seeming impossibilities, faith holds fast to the truth of God's Word over and above the facts.

As Pastor Stan stepped to the pulpit to begin his sermon he announced that I had received a bad report from the doctor and that at the close of the service, the church would be praying for me. After the service I went to the altar and several of my friends came and laid hands on me according to Mark 16:17, believers shall "...lay hands on the sick, and they shall recover." They anointed me with oil and prayed for the healing of my body according to James 5:14. I remember Donnie Wood, who had been healed of cancer some twenty years earlier, prayed over me. It has been my experience, and I believe I am in accordance with Scripture to have only those who believe in healing to lay their hands on you and pray. I knew I didn't want anyone who believed otherwise to pray for me.

Some of the ladies from the church stayed and continued to pray. I remember one friend, Jo Ann Miller, said to me, "Deborah, when I heard Pastor Stan say you had received a bad report, I thought, *Oh no, not Deborah.*"

I found myself consoling her. She was genuinely hurting for me. I told her, "Jo Ann, it's going to be alright." And I truly believed that it would be.

I was still discovering all the wonderful truths in God's Word concerning healing, but I was beginning to operate in the mustard-seed of faith that I had by speaking confidently about what the Word says instead of what the doctor said. I was learning to receive Jesus as my Healer, and I was learning to receive the healing that He had purchased for me 2,000 years ago.

I had always found it easy to believe that when I received Christ as my Savior He came into my heart and delivered me from all my sins. I decided it was better to believe that He also delivered me from sickness and disease than to disbelieve and wonder if healing would really come. Either the Bible is true or it isn't. Either we believe the Bible or we don't. If the Bible says it, I believe it!

For most, including me, *believing* is not the hard part where healing is concerned; it's *receiving* that often stumps us. James gives us the remedy for the receiving in 1:22,

where he instructs us to "...be doers of the word, and not hearers only...."

The following night I went back to Christ Church for prayer with three men known as "The Three J's": Jim, Jack, and John…and of course, Jesus. The Three J's had prayed every Monday night by appointment for more than twenty years. These men knew some things about prayer, and, about results. Brother Jim had some specific words to speak over me that night. What he said bore witness with what was in my heart, but what I had never put into words. He said, "I am not finished with you. I have a great work to do in you and I am going to show you My great power."

His words, I believe inspired by the Holy Spirit, lifted me up and bolstered my faith. I cannot describe how I felt as I drove home that night, saturated in the peace and presence of God. It was amazing for me to realize that the God of Abraham, Isaac, and Jacob had spoken into my life at a time when I needed Him the most.

He's the Way Maker

Every step of my journey was truly a step of faith. Not only was I believing God for the healing of my body, but I was also depending upon Him for help on the financial side. As anyone can imagine, surgery and numerous radiation treatments were going to add up. Following the consultation with Dr. Spaw, Charlie and I began to pray and believe God to provide a way for us to obtain insurance coverage. We had made arrangements to have the second surgery on April 12, one month from the consultation date; however, this was contingent upon our having insurance.

God is a God of the miraculous! He makes a way where there is no way and He is always right on time. My sister Peggy bumped into a long-time acquaintance who "just happened" to work for the Governor of Tennessee. This friend worked in the legislative department and could help me obtain the state insurance provider for those considered uninsurable. That described me to a tee. What insurance carrier would choose to insure someone diagnosed with a deadly disease? Peggy's friend and our pastor's brother-in-law, Bob Clement, who was also our congressman, proved to be the divine connection God used to make a way for me. Bob's step-son, Jeff, is a friend of Charlie's and mine. When he heard the report of breast cancer and no insurance, he was devastated. He phoned Bob, and between them and a client of my sister's who worked for the state legislative department, I was able to receive Tenn Care, the state's insurance program for those who are uninsurable. Another friend was able to obtain a letter from State Farm stating that I was indeed "uninsurable," proof of which was required to receive Tenn Care. Once everything was in order, all I had to do was pay a premium every month. Isn't God great?!

At the same time God was working out details with the insurance, He was also preparing another divine encounter. Nancy Alcorn, president of Mercy Ministries of America, was one of our catering customers. One afternoon the home was holding a meeting for which we were providing the box lunches. I had a chance to visit with Nancy that day. She asked me some pointed questions to help me locate exactly where I was, where I needed to be, and what I needed to do to get there. "Have you been reading God's Word and what it says about healing?" Nancy asked.

I honestly hadn't. "No" I told her, and proceeded to make one excuse after the other as to why not. It had only been a few days since we had received word about the cancer and, after all, I was busy.

Make a note, that kind of thinking will never get anyone healed. We must give the Word of God *first place* in our lives if we want to experience the promises Jesus purchased at Calvary. Any excuse that takes the place of God's Word is a lie from Satan! The Bible tells us that the devil is the father of lies. His job is to kill, steal, and destroy (John 10:10), and he was working 24/7 on me trying to convince me that I didn't have time to read healing scriptures.

Truthfully, my life was so busy with home responsibilities, our catering business, and church obligations that I really had very little time on my hands to sit and read my Bible, let alone soak in the Word on healing. I could see that if I was serious about obtaining my healing, I was going to have to make some major adjustments in how I spent my time. With surgery only four weeks away, every moment counted.

Keep in mind I really had no basis for believing I would be healed other than the dream God gave me. My hope stemmed from a *desire* to be healed, but dear friends, that is not enough. If we are going to stand on the Word of God then we must do whatever it takes to build His Word inside of us, laying a firm foundation on which to stand. I didn't *want* to believe the doctor's report; I didn't *want* to lose excessive amounts of weight and be sick and helpless like Daddy. But what we want or don't want is of no consequence. We can want all day and that doesn't cause what we want to happen. I can park myself in my garage but that is not going to make me a car. Hope is necessary and prayer is vital, but neither one produces faith. Hoping and praying simply produce hoping and praying for something we have no proof of receiving. The Word of God planted in our heart is the only substance that will produce faith, and faith is the only way to obtain the promises of God.

Faith was definitely the key on two occasions for individuals in Mark 5. Notice the account of Jairus, a man whose daughter was on the verge of death.

> **Now when Jesus had crossed over again by boat to the other side, a great multitude gathered to Him; and He was by the sea.**
>
> **And behold, one of the rulers of the synagogue came, Jairus by name. And when he saw Him, he fell at His feet and begged Him earnestly, saying, "My little daughter lies at the point of death. Come and lay Your hands on her, that she may be healed, and she will live."**
>
> **So Jesus went with him, and a great multitude followed Him and thronged Him.**

Mark 5:21–24

In the middle of Jesus' journey to this man's house, the faith of one woman amidst the pressing crowd drew His attention away long enough for another miracle to take place.

Now a certain woman had a flow of blood for twelve years, and had suffered many things from many physicians. She had spent all that she had and was no better, but rather grew worse.

When she heard about Jesus, she came behind Him in the crowd and touched His garment; for she said, "If only I may touch His clothes, I shall be made well."

. Immediately the fountain of her blood was dried up, and she felt in her body that she was healed of the affliction.

And Jesus, immediately knowing in Himself that power had gone out of Him, turned around in the crowd and said, "Who touched My clothes?"

But His disciples said to Him, "You see the multitude thronging You, and You say, 'Who touched Me?' "

And He looked around to see her who had done this thing.

But the woman, fearing and trembling, knowing what had happened to her, came and fell down before Him and told Him the whole truth.

And He said to her, "Daughter, *your* faith has made you well. Go in peace, and be healed of your affliction."

Mark 5:25–34, italics added

While He was still speaking, some came from the ruler of the synagogue's house who said, "Your daughter is dead. Why trouble the Teacher any further?"

As soon as Jesus heard the word that was spoken, He said to the ruler of the synagogue, "Do not be afraid; only *believe.*"

And He permitted no one to follow Him except Peter, James, and John the brother of James.

Then He came to the house of the ruler of the synagogue, and saw a tumult and those who wept and wailed loudly.

33

When He came in, He said to them, "Why make this commotion and weep? The child is not dead, but sleeping."

And they ridiculed Him. But when He had put them all outside, He took the father and the mother of the child, and those who were with Him, and entered where the child was lying.

Then He took the child by the hand, and said to her, "Talitha, cumi," which is translated, "Little girl, I say to you, arise."

Immediately the girl arose and walked, for she was twelve years of age. And they were overcome with great amazement.

Mark 5:35–42, italics added

Huge crowds gathered around Jesus the moment He stepped out of the boat after having crossed from the other side of the sea. People were pushing and shoving their way passed one another to get to Him. Jairus was an important man, a ruler of the synagogue, I suppose like the mayor of a city in comparison. Even so, the people didn't part for him; he had to make his way through the crowds just like anyone else. When he finally got to Jesus, the Bible says he fell at His feet and earnestly begged Him to come and lay His hands on his little girl that she might be healed and live.

Jairus didn't care what the people thought; he was desperate. His family had a need and he was going to do whatever it took to see that the need was met. This is the kind of bulldog determination you have to have about your healing. When it's you or someone you love and care about who needs a touch from God, you will do whatever it takes regardless of what others think.

The story was the same with the woman with the issue of blood. Her *faith* caused her to press through every obstacle in her path. Her faith caused her to stretch out her hand with the expectation that when she touched only the hem of Jesus' garment, she would be healed. Her faith was strong enough to stop Jesus in His tracks, when He was fully aware that power had gone out of Him—power to heal anyone who would believe. And heal it did. The woman, who had suffered twelve years even at the hands of the most well trained physicians of the day, sensed her flow of blood dry up instantly. If we want the results these scriptural examples of faith had, we must be willing to do whatever it takes, regardless of the opinions of man.

Every time I saw Nancy Alcorn, she asked me if I had read *Christ the Healer* by F. F. Bosworth.

"No, not yet," I told her.

Her reply was always the same: "You need to."

She gave me some small, pocket-size books by Charles Capps, Brother Kenneth Copeland, and Brother Kenneth E. Hagin to read.

35

All the books were on healing. She also told me that she, her staff, and the girls at Mercy Ministries wanted to pray for me. A day later, Charlie and I spent the morning at the ministry where they laid hands on me, anointed me with oil, and prayed for my healing. I felt the Lord's love and compassion for me flowing through the hearts, hands and prayers of those lovely women that day. Yet, even with all they did, I still had not done my part. I allowed Satan to convince me that I didn't have time to read *Christ the Healer*, the book Nancy so strongly urged me to read. *I didn't even have the book, and I certainly didn't have time to go find it*, I thought, again giving in to the enemy's lies.

Did you know the Bible says, "My people are destroyed for lack of knowledge"? I definitely did not want to become a casualty based on my lack of knowledge of God's Word. In His mercy, God provided me with the book that would help establish me in His Word on healing. As I delivered a box lunch order to Mercy Ministries one day, a staff member asked me how I was doing. I tried to keep the conversation light with pleasant chit-chat, but that didn't last long. This woman looked through my defensive exterior right into my heart. As I prepared to leave, she said to me with great conviction, "Deborah, we are all believing that you are healed by the stripes of Jesus."

The woman walked me to the Mercy Ministries library, graciously furnished by Kenneth and Gloria Copeland with a wealth of Word-based material. There I found it: F. F. Bosworth's book, *Christ the*

Healer. "Take it," she said smiling from ear to ear. "It just arrived yesterday." Again, God was right on time, and He had made sure that I was in the right place at the right time.

I recall as I left and sat down in my vehicle, I said to myself, "Deborah, these people—some of whom you've just met—are believing you are healed, but you aren't believing it for yourself."

Wonderful people of faith could pray and believe for me, but God expected *me* to believe and receive for myself. He knew what was up ahead and how important it was for me to use this time to prepare myself; to get myself in a position to receive the healing He had provided for me. The Scriptures tell us that Jesus could do no mighty work in His hometown of Nazareth, except lay His hands on a few sick folks…because of their *unbelief* (Mark 6:5–6).

Hebrews 11:6, says, "…without *faith* it is impossible to please Him…" (italics added). God needed *my* faith, and my excuses were running out.

The Word of God says:

> **My son, *attend* to my words; *incline thine ear* unto my sayings.**
>
> **Let them not depart from thine eyes; *keep them* in the midst of thine heart.**
>
> **For *they are life* unto those that find them, *and health* to all their flesh.**

Proverbs 4:20–22, italics added

God had provided me with believing people of prayer, countless books, Sister Gloria Copeland's Healing School tapes, and above all that, His own Word. What more could He do? He tells us that life and death are set before *us*, and that *we* are to choose. He even gives us a hint about the right choice; He tells us to choose *life* (Deuteronomy 30:19–20). It's like taking an open book test. If we do as the Word instructs, we cannot fail!

God has a will, and it's for all of His children to walk in the divine health and healing He provided through His Son, Jesus Christ. Every good and perfect gift comes from God (James 1:17). God is a good God who gives good gifts to His children, and healing is part of the package! What earthly parent would want his or her child sick? Certainly only a parent with no love or concern for his child. How much more does our heavenly Father desire for us to be well? God has done His part regarding healing, and we must do ours. Our part is to read His Word, to plant His truth in our heart, to speak in agreement with what His Word says is ours, and to walk in the rich benefits He has provided for us.

He is Jehovah – jireh: the Lord will provide!

He is Jehovah – rapha: the Lord thy physician or the Lord that healeth!

Finally, I understood that I had a part to play in my healing that went beyond my *desire* to be healed. I began to carve out time to read the Word of God. I started reading the pocket books Nancy had given me about healing. Then, I took another step and looked up healing scriptures in my Bible, scriptures such as: Hosea 4:6, Luke 6:45, Proverbs 4:20, First Peter 2:24 and others.

Meditate in the Word Day and Night

One day as I was studying the Scriptures, I asked the Lord, "How will I ever get enough faith to believe for my healing?"

His response was clear and direct. "Meditate in the Word day and night," He told me.

Charlie and I set out to do just that. Every morning as soon as our feet hit the floor, we were either in the Word, listening to Sister Copeland's Healing School tapes, or listening to Brother and Sister Copeland's Praise Healing tapes where healing scriptures are spoken between praise songs and the reading of the Word. We also took a black Sharpie and wrote out healing scriptures on the bathroom mirror and on yellow legal pads—about two scriptures to a page—and taped them all over our kitchen since that is where we spent most of our time. We were *attending* to the Word, *keeping it before our eyes*, as Proverbs 4:20–21 say to do. Whatever we keep before our eyes and hear with our ears will work its way into our heart and eventually be spoken out of our mouth. Luke 6:45 says, "…out of the abundance of the heart his (the) mouth speaks." Therefore, whatever is in our heart in abundance is what we will say. If we are obsessed with our job, our house, our grandchildren, or whatever, that is what is going to come out of our mouth.

This total immersion in the Word of God was all very new to us. Initially, I didn't notice much of a change. In fact, the first week we were feeding on the tapes and books I happened to take a box lunch order to Patty and Cecil Kemp's office. Patty and Cecil are acquaintances. They are faith filled, Word-walking, caring people. They actually gave us enough catering business in the beginning to help our business grow, and truly they have the gift of encouragement. They kept me on their "in house" e-mail and prayed for me every day. I visited their office three or four times a week to deliver box lunches, and Cecil always said the same thing. He asked me every time how I was feeling. "Well," I would reply, "the doctor said...." And every time he would look at me and say, "No! Deborah you are healed by the stripes of Jesus."

I'd stop myself and think, *Okay, I can do this.* I still didn't have the revelation that He *took* my sicknesses and *carried* my pains, and that by His stripes I *had been*—past tense—healed.

Romans 10:17 says, "So then faith cometh by hearing, and hearing by the word of God."

It takes hearing and hearing the Word before that Word is planted in our hearts and faith begins to grow to the point that the Word comes out of our mouth. We have to know the Word before we can believe it or have faith in it, because we can't believe in something we don't know anything about.

By the end of the second week, we had listened to Sister Gloria's Healing School tapes enough that I could tell you what she was going to say next. I remember one day my sister called and was crying and upset over a situation in her life. It was about 9:30 in the morning and I realized she was on a cell phone. "Where are you?" I asked. "Aren't you calling from work?"

No, she wasn't, she was on her way over to our house.

"Lord," I said, "I don't have time for this. I am trying to make box lunches for an order and I am so busy."

We should never be too busy for the lessons God wants to teach us, and He had other plans for me at that moment.

My sister often came to our house for lunch, and when she came, Sister Gloria's tapes kept right on playing. We didn't turn the tapes off just because someone came over; we had work to do, and believe me, when it's a matter of life and death you had better be willing to work. The Word of God doesn't just come and stick to you. You have to go after the Word and prepare your heart to take it in and receive it.

When my sister arrived, she was crying and clearly upset about some choices she had made. She began to tell me all about her troubles and about how badly she felt. I looked at her and said rather sternly, "Do you not think I could just sit here in this kitchen and feel sorry for myself?" All the while Sister Copeland's tape was playing in the background. I knew I wasn't getting through to her, but one thing was certain, she knew she wasn't going to get any sympathy from me.

As she got up to leave, I turned and very abruptly told her, "I told you that if you would resist the enemy that he would flee from you."

Startled, she paid me the greatest compliment she could have given me: "You sound just like Gloria Copeland," she said.

That was it: the turning point! In an instant, I realized this Word was getting into my heart. I wasn't wasting time or just going through the motions of some rote memory exercise. The living Word of God was being planted in my heart to the point it was now coming out of my mouth instinctively. Thank you Lord, I had turned another corner on the road to victory!

Chapter 4

The Barrier of Unforgiveness

And when ye stand praying, forgive, if ye have ought against any: that your Father also which is in heaven may forgive you your trespasses.

Mark 11:25

Healing and forgiveness go hand in hand. If you have been standing for healing in your body and the results don't seem to be coming, check "inside" and see if there is something in your heart that doesn't belong there. Do you have "ought" against someone? Against God? Even against yourself? If so, that unforgiveness could be the barrier standing between you and your healing.

As I continued to study the Word, God revealed a powerful truth to me about unforgiveness. The Bible tells us: "Confess your trespasses to one another, and pray for one another, *that you may be healed.* The effective, fervent prayer of a righteous man avails much" (James 5:16, italics added).

A righteous man is one who is in right standing with God. If we have unforgiveness in our heart toward a brother, sister, or anyone else, then the Bible says neither will God forgive us (Mark 11:26). If God hasn't forgiven us, then we are not in right standing with Him.

I didn't have to dig too deep to find the unforgiveness I was carrying in my heart against my sister Peggy. I had always loved Peggy, but I honestly didn't like her. I thought she was a phony. The Bible says, "The entrance of *his* word gives light…" (Psalm 119:130), and when the light of the Word shone in this area of my life, I saw my error and knew I would need to confess this sin to my sister and forgive her. I called her on the phone after returning home from a retreat and told her how I felt. I asked her to forgive me for not believing the best about her and for holding these feelings against her in my heart. She graciously forgave me and our relationship was restored.

The Spirit of Offense

Offense is often the seed that, given the right environment, will take root in our heart and grow into unforgiveness. We should do everything possible to avoid becoming offended. Getting our feelings hurt and being touchy or resentful opens the door wide to whatever Satan wants to do.

Throughout this journey, I searched my heart many times. I prayed and asked God to reveal to me if I was harboring unforgiveness toward anyone. I repented of everything I could think of, and anything I had done unknowingly that might hinder God from moving in my life. I know that sometimes our flesh wants to be angry and hold a grudge, especially when someone really has done us wrong. But Jesus forgave us didn't He? We have to look at every situation from God's perspective, not our own. His thoughts are not our thoughts and our ways are not His ways (Isaiah 55:8). The more we feed on His Word, the more like Him we will become until our thinking is renewed according to Romans 12:2, and we have the mind of Christ (1 Corinthians 2:16).

The Word of God helped me to keep my heart clear of the clutter of offense and unforgiveness, which are sins. God's plan was too important for me to give the enemy so much as one inch. I was determined that no barrier was going to come between my healing and me, because my life depended upon it.

A Second Opinion

Charlie and I had been listening to tapes and studying God's Word for almost two weeks before we went to Vanderbilt Breast Center for a second opinion. Brother Jim, one of the gentlemen who prayed for me at church, had encouraged me to have a second opinion based on a situation he had read about in the newspaper. A woman in our area had been diagnosed with breast cancer and had both breasts removed, only to find out afterward that she had been misdiagnosed.

We were scheduled with Dr. Reynolds on Wednesday morning, March 27 for the second opinion. He had been highly recommended by a cousin of mine who had lost her breast to cancer some fifteen years ago at that time. We found Dr. Reynolds to be very pleasant. He examined me and talked with us for what I thought was a much longer time than a doctor would usually take, especially one who knows he is not the primary physician.

His prognosis was this: he agreed with Dr. Spaw that because cancer cells were left all around the edge of the tumor, that going back into surgery to remove more breast tissue would help insure that all the "feelers" would be removed. At the same time they removed the "feelers" he agreed that they should also remove the lymph nodes and check them.

While we were there, I asked Dr. Reynolds if his pathologist could look at the reports and biopsies that we had brought with us. He told us they wouldn't have time to look at them that day, "but with your positive attitude," he said optimistically, "you will be fine."

Before we left the office, Dr. Reynolds's nurse invited me to a support group meeting. She had started the group to listen to and comfort other women with breast cancer. I thought I would test the waters a bit, so I nonchalantly mentioned something about trusting God to help me through this ordeal. I don't know how to describe the look on her face any other way than to say she looked at me as if I had a third eyeball! (Some people say more with actions than with words.)

I graciously told her that I appreciated her invitation to the support group, but that I was not going to come to a pity party. I am sure some women benefit from this type of consoling, but I knew the only support I needed would come from studying and *receiving* God's Word concerning healing. We left Dr. Reynolds's office with such peace—the peace that passes understanding (Philippians 4:7).

Changed by the Word

The Word of God was changing me from the inside out. When you study God's Word, you know that you know that you know God says what He means and means what He says. Second Timothy 3:16 says that *all* Scripture—every printed word in the Bible—is the inspired Word of God. The Bible also says that the Word of God is truth (John 17:17), and that God is not a man that he should lie (Numbers 23:19). The more Charlie and I saturated ourselves with His Word—His truth—the more we began to receive it into our hearts. Out of the abundance of the heart, the mouth speaks, and this same truth began spewing out of our mouths. Every time someone asked me how I felt, I told them, "I am healed by the stripes of Jesus" (1 Peter 2:24).

I recall when I was first diagnosed, Charlie went to his Wednesday morning prayer breakfast and asked the men there to pray specifically for my healing. He told them that God's will is that I be well, and if they couldn't pray in line with that, then he didn't want them to pray at all. They stared at him in shock—as if he had just landed from another planet. *How arrogant,* some thought. But Charlie's attitude was one of neither pride nor arrogance. His words were not meant to be condemning of anyone who didn't believe as we did. We had simply dug deep enough into the Word to see for ourselves the truth about God's will concerning healing.

When unbelief is confronted by truth, it's not the truth that will bend; it's the unbelief that will be overturned. The bold confidence we had concerning the Word wasn't because we were anything special. God is no respecter of persons, but He is a respecter of His Word. His Word was changing us. As we attended to the Word and believed it, we began to receive tangible results!

Believing and Receiving

Matthew 21:22 says, "And whatever things you ask in prayer, *believing*, you will *receive*."

So Jesus answered and said to them, "Have faith in God.

"For assuredly, I say to you, whoever says to this mountain, 'Be removed and be cast into the sea,' and does not doubt in his heart, but believes that those things he says will come to pass, he will have whatever he says.

"Therefore I say to you, whatever things you ask when you pray, *believe* that you *receive* them, and you will have them."

Mark 11:22–24

Does *"whatever things you ask in prayer"* include healing from sickness in your body? Then *receive* Jesus as your Healer!

John 14:13–14 says, "And whatever you ask in My name, that I will do, that the Father may be glorified in the Son. If you ask anything in My name, I will do it."

Do *"whatever you ask in My name"* and *"if you ask anything in My name"* include healing from sickness in your body? Then *receive* Jesus as your Healer!

John 15:7 tells us, "If you abide in Me, and My words abide in you, you will ask what you desire, and it shall be done for you."

Does *"you will ask what you desire"* include healing from sickness in your body? Then *receive* Jesus as your Healer!

First John 3:22 says, "And whatever we ask we receive from Him, because we keep His commandments and do those things that are pleasing in His sight."

Does *"whatever we ask"* include healing from sickness in your body? Then *receive* Jesus as your Healer, for He is no respecter of persons; what He does for one, He will do for all, "only believe!"

He Is Willing

A leper came to Jesus for healing, saying, "Lord, if you are willing, you can make me clean." In other words, "I know you can heal me, but do you *want* to heal me; are you willing?"

Jesus answered him, "I am willing; be cleansed" (Matthew 8:2–3).

It is one thing to know that God *can* heal, but it is another thing to know that He *is willing* to heal.

Jesus came to do the Father's will. If healing was not God's will for all, and Jesus "went about doing good and healing *all*" then He would have been doing things against the Father's will. Jesus said, "He who has seen Me has seen the Father" (John 14:9).

If you have any question that healing is God's will for all, including you, I want to eliminate every ounce of doubt. Through God's Word, I am going to transform your thinking until you know without a doubt that it is God's will for you to be well. The authority of God's Word will cause you to confidently believe that not only is He *able* to heal you, but He is also *willing* to heal you.

We must first establish that God is not the author of sickness and disease. James 1:17 says, "Every good gift…comes from above." Sickness and disease are not good. God doesn't have any sickness or disease, so He couldn't be the one to give it. We quoted a portion of Acts 10:38 earlier, which says, "…God anointed Jesus of Nazareth with the Holy Spirit and with power, who went about doing good and healing all who were *oppressed by the devil*, for God was with Him."

It is clear to see the source of sickness and disease; they come right from the pit of hell.

The Scriptures tell us in Psalm 91:15–16, "He shall call upon Me, and I will answer him; I will be with him in trouble; I will deliver him and honor him. With long life *(length of days)* I will satisfy him, And show him My salvation." God's will is for us to enjoy a long, satisfying life, free from the bondage of our enemy, Satan.

Smith Wigglesworth (1859–1947), was a plumber in England, who, once baptized in the Holy Spirit, became a fiery preacher with a ministry marked by incredible healings, miracles, and even numerous documented accounts of people being raised from the dead. A man who learned the secret of the power of God's Word, Wigglesworth is quoted as saying, "I understand God by His Word. I cannot understand God by impressions or feelings. I cannot get to know God by sentiment. I can only know Him by His Word."[1]

It is dangerous to be governed by our feelings. Hebrews 11:1 says, "Now faith is the substance of things hoped for, the evidence of things not seen."

Our feelings can tell us our body doesn't feel well, our condition hasn't changed, and the symptoms are still there, but what does faith say? Faith says we are to believe and say what the Word says: that we have been healed by the stripes of Jesus. Second Corinthians 5:7 instructs us to, "...walk by faith, not by sight." When we see

---

[1] Albert Hibbert, *Smith Wigglesworth – The Secret of His Power* (Tulsa: Harrison House, 1982), 32.

ourselves through the eye of faith, we see ourselves healed, whole, and perfectly well.

We read in Luke 6:17–19:

> **And He came down with them and stood on a level place with a crowd of His disciples and a great multitude of people from all Judea and Jerusalem, and from the seacoast of Tyre and Sidon, who came to hear Him and be healed of their diseases, as well as those who were tormented with unclean spirits. And they were healed. And the whole multitude sought to touch Him, for power went out from Him and healed them all.**

Are you beginning to see it? The cure for unbelief is teaching, preaching, and the demonstration of healing. Jesus may have corrected people for their unbelief, but He never condemned them. He simply kept giving them the truth.

If it be Thy Will

One Saturday morning I had gone to Christ Church to set up a luncheon for their "Understanding God and His Covenants" class. The teacher of the class, Beverly Robbins, knew of the report I had been given, and asked me if I would like to share it with the class counselors so that they could pray. I told her of course I would.

Charlie and I had taken this class several years ago and had served as counselors. We knew what dedication to the Lord this role required. I shared the doctor's report with these individuals and asked them to pray for my healing, specifically instructing them *not to pray*, "If it be thy will." I realized this would be a new concept to some, and explained that I understood some of them might not be able to pray that way. If they couldn't, I said it was alright, but if they could, I told them I would appreciate their prayers.

Even for some reading these pages, you might be wondering why I would make an issue out of people—godly, praying people—praying "if it be thy will." If it were not such a common practice, I wouldn't have had the need to address it. Many people truly believe that it is scriptural to pray, "if it be thy will" concerning healing. But this way of praying is nothing more than a manmade tradition. The Bible says that the traditions of man make the Word of God of no effect (Matthew 15:6). *The Amplified Bible* reads this way: "So for the sake of your tradition (the rules handed down by your forefathers), you have set aside the Word of God, depriving it of force and authority and making it of no effect."

The parallel passage in the Book of Mark reads:

> **He answered and said to them, "Well did Isaiah prophesy of you hypocrites, as it is written:**
>
> **"This people honors Me with their lips, But their heart is far from Me. And in vain**

they worship Me, Teaching as doctrines the commandments of men.

"For laying aside the commandment of God, you hold the tradition of men—the washing of pitchers and cups, and many other such things you do."

And He said to them, "All too well you reject the commandment of God, that you may keep your tradition.

"For Moses said, 'Honor your father and your mother'; and, 'He who curses father or mother, let him be put to death.'

"But you say, 'If a man says to his father or mother, "Whatever profit you might have received from me is Corban"—'(that is, a gift to God),'

"then you no longer let him do anything for his father or his mother,

"making the word of God of no effect through your tradition which you have handed down. And many such things you do."

Mark 7:6–13

We are to be doers of the Word and not hearers only. Faith without works or corresponding action is dead. Charlie and I believed that getting the Word of God in our hearts produced faith, and speaking it out of our mouth was the corresponding action. Any time and every time anyone delicately patted me on the back and asked, "Honey, how are you feeling?" I would always respond, "I am healed by the stripes of Jesus." But this didn't happen overnight. I grew in my knowledge and understanding of God's promises concerning healing, and began to line my mouth up with the Word after my initial encounters with Patty and Cecil Kemp, and after I had fed on the Scriptures for a number of weeks.

A Night of Breakthrough

Patty and Cecil were instrumental in our lives. They were not only customers, but also true friends. They were acquainted with two older sisters in the Lord who went about preaching the Word—women who would have a profound impact on our lives. Tuesday night, March 26, the night before I saw Dr. Reynolds for the second opinion, Patty and Cecil had invited Charlie and me to their home to share in a night of teaching and fellowship with Christian friends, as well as to cater the desserts and coffee after the meeting. I had gladly accepted the invitation with anticipation. I couldn't quite put my finger on it, but somehow I knew there was something different about these women who would be sharing the Word that night.

Charlie and I arrived at their home and began preparing the desserts for the fellowship. I remember standing at the kitchen island when Cecil came in the side door of their home and into the kitchen. As I was plating the desserts, he walked behind me, stood by my left shoulder and said, "Deborah, how are you?"

I turned to look at him in the eye and said with confident assurance, "Cecil, I am a healed woman by the stripes of Jesus."

A great big smile spread across his face. You see, he knew all that I had been doing had become real to me. The seeds of faith I had been sowing had finally taken root in my heart. The Scriptures say that whatever we sow, that we will also reap (Galatians 6:7). Charlie and I had been sowing "Word seeds" and our harvest was coming in!

Jesus always used simple illustrations in His teachings, examples that people could relate to such as farming. What if a farmer said, "I really want a big harvest this year. I'm counting on big, beautiful ears of corn, the biggest crop I have ever had"? But when you asked him how much seed he planted, his corn seeds were still in the bag on his front porch. That farmer is not going to reap a crop. He's not going to reap anything.

That is ridiculous, some might think. Yes, it is. It is so ridiculous because we do it all the time in many areas of our lives. We beg and plead with God that we want this possession, or that blessing, but we haven't planted any seed in order to reap what we desire. The simple truth is: no seed, no harvest.

Regarding healing, when our eyes are on our body and our mind is occupied with our symptoms more than with God's Word, we have the wrong kind of seed in the ground. We desire a harvest of health and healing, but in the ground we've sown seeds of doubt and unbelief. We are trying to produce a certain kind of crop from a different type of seed.

Just as in the natural it is impossible to sow corn and reap wheat, in the spirit realm we cannot plant seeds of doubt in our heart and expect to reap health and life. Our symptoms may point to death, but God's Word points to life! We've got to keep our eyes on the Author and the Finisher of our faith, Jesus! We can't look in the opposite direction at the same time. After we have planted our seed, by faith we believe it is growing, even before we see the harvest. Remember, faith is the *substance* of things hoped for, the *evidence* of things *not seen.*

In Christ, we have perfect evidence of faith. Believing what God says and seeing the way He sees—through the eyes of faith—will produce a harvest of whatever it is we are believing. God has given us sixty-six bags of seed! We must take those "Word seeds" and bombard our heart with them.

See yourself well! Recognize where you are today and accept the challenge and the responsibility to put the Word first place in your life. You will be so thankful you chose to take God at His Word as you begin to reap a harvest of healing in your body.

That night at Patty and Cecil's home there were about seventeen of us gathered to hear Sister Dora preach. Most were staff from Christ Church and were also our friends. We all packed into the living room. Patty sat on the piano bench and I was across the room in a chair.

As sister Dora ministered the Word, she began to talk about healing. "I really don't know why I am telling you all this," she said, surprised. My eyes darted across the room to where Patty sat; tears were rolling down her face as she looked at me. Patty and Cecil had been walking this "faith walk" for years, and they wanted so badly for Charlie and me to grab hold of the healing promises of God. Just as Charlie and I have, I'm sure they saw friends and family die from this deadly disease, not knowing that Jesus bore all sickness and disease for us at Calvary.

After Sister Dora finished preaching, she began to call different people forward to speak directly into their lives. This was an area Charlie and I had not grown in, and we were somewhat hesitant about what was happening. I watched as the individuals began to "fall out." *What have we gotten ourselves into?* I thought. I just didn't know about this "falling out stuff." Were they being pushed, manipulated, or what? I was asking myself *Why did I come tonight? She's going to start calling everyone up there and then she's going to push them down.* The more I thought about what might happen, the more miserable I grew. I wanted to be anywhere but in that living room.

Do you know Satan is a liar and a thief? He did his very best that night to try to rob me of the blessing God had planned for me.

Perhaps Patty and Cecil sensed the battle going on in my mind and began to pray, because all of a sudden right up out of my spirit came, "No! God, I want all that You have for me tonight...*everything!*"

Sure enough, just then she called Charlie out. She spoke over him and barely touched him on the forehead and he fell to the floor under the power of God. Then, I heard my name and made my way to the front of the room. I don't have any recollection of what Sister Dora said, but I do remember how the tip of her finger touched me ever so lightly and I, too, fell under the power of God. I lay there thirty minutes, shaking all over. I tried to get up, but couldn't. It was as if God was saying, "No, I'm not finished with you yet." Brother Jim had prophesied these same words over me right after I had been diagnosed.

As I lay there on the floor, another woman, Sister Clara, came over and knelt down beside me. Just like Sister Dora, she had no idea that I had been given a bad report from the doctor. She began to wave her hands over my chest area and said over and over again, "There is something going on here."

Finally, the Lord allowed me to get up. Carol Bryant, a friend from Christ Church, came over to help me. She literally had to carry me because I was so drunk in the Spirit I couldn't stand up or walk by myself. The Bible says we are not to be drunk with wine...but to be *filled with the Spirit* just as the 120 were on the Day of Pentecost, and as believers are continually filled to this day (Ephesians 5:18, Acts 2:1–21). Carol sat me down in a chair. I was still so weak I couldn't even hold my arms up. What a glorious night—one I'm glad God planned for me!

Tonight was a night of breakthrough for me. Charlie and I had forged through many crossroads, maneuvered past roadblocks, and broken through significant barriers of unbelief and unforgiveness. The Holy Spirit was guiding us magnificently down a path of healing, and the best was yet to come!

Chapter 5

Fulfillment of the Promise

As the surgery date approached, Charlie and I continued to feed on God's Word and fill our days with catering clients. At Christ Church we were preparing to host our annual Word and Spirit Conference, and I had been given the position of food coordinator. I never actually wanted to cater this event; I only wanted to give my time and energies as an offering to the Lord.

I reported to Joy Wright, a lovely woman on staff at Christ Church. One afternoon during a planning meeting for the conference, Joy asked me when I was going to have the surgery. "You don't really want to know," I told her. But she persisted in asking. (I just knew she would all but keel over if I told her the surgery was scheduled on Friday, just two days before the conference began on Sunday!)

I finally told her that the surgery was on Friday.

"Oh," she said, "the Friday after the conference."

"No, the Friday before."

I was right; she nearly fainted.

"I have everything under control," I told her.

Volunteers were lined up. They were all faithful people who loved serving the Lord. I could see that Joy had her doubts, but I did my best to reassure her that everything would be covered.

A Surprise Attack

With the surgery only five days away, an unexpected turn of events required me to make an emergency visit to the oral surgeon. An infection in the gum of my left jaw had to be cleared up at once or the breast surgery could not be performed. Just what I needed: an abscess, three teeth extracted, and a mouth *full* of stitches!

The dentist instructed me to make sure to tell the doctors that I had had oral surgery and that the stitches were still in place. He didn't want the stitches to be broken while the anesthesia was being administered.

Normally something like this might have shaken me up, but such a peace rested on me. I knew that I knew God's Word was working in my body, driving out the cancer, and restoring me to health. The same healing power that whipped cancer would also eradicate any underlying infection and heal my mouth and gum tissue. No surprise attack of the enemy was going to discourage me or deter my faith and get me into fear. Charlie and I had come too far. We set our faces like flint, and kept our focus on the finish line.

Standing on the Word

I recall one particular day before the second surgery; a young man selling candy came to the front door of our home. His head hung low as he began to recite a little speech about what he was selling to earn money toward a trip his church was taking. I had such compassion on him as I listened. I could see he had no confidence in himself.

I told him, "Honey, don't hold your head down low. Everywhere you go tonight know that God will go before you to prepare the hearts of those you are to see."

Then to his surprise, I sat down and took my shoes off to show him the pieces of paper that I had written healing scriptures on and taped to the soles of my shoes. I had reminded God of His promises to me and told him that I was literally standing on His Word. I told this young man that he, too, could trust God to help him sell his candy.

"You're the second person who has talked to me about God tonight," he told me, and he strutted away with newfound confidence.

I was grateful that God had allowed me to witness His goodness to this young man. God told us in Isaiah 55:11, "So shall My Word be that goes forth from My mouth, it shall not return to me void, but it shall accomplish what I please, and shall prosper in the thing for which I sent it."

I believed that the power in God's Word had been sent forth to heal me, and it was prospering!

The Chastisement of Our Peace

Friday, April 12 finally arrived. Charlie and I awoke at 4:00 A.M., and headed for the Baptist Hospital Outpatient an hour later to make our scheduled appointment time of 5:30 A.M. There was something so different about this trip to the hospital. When I had visited the Nashville Surgical Center Outpatient facility to have the lump removed from my breast, I had no idea what would follow. This time I knew exactly what was in store, yet I had more peace than I did the first visit. Something was different. *I* was different. The Word of God planted in my heart had changed me. I was bolder, stronger, more confident, and more adamant than ever that Jesus was my Healer.

As we neared the downtown area where the Baptist Hospital was located, I noticed Charlie growing unusually quiet. "I need to ask you something," he said, breaking the silence.

In my spirit I knew what he was going to say. I could sense that he did not want to sound doubtful in any way, especially at a time like this, and after we had worked so hard to build faith in our hearts. Charlie's words were carefully chosen and softly spoken. "Deborah," he said, "you know how sometimes the family member has to make decisions for the patient?"

"Yes, Charlie, that does happen sometimes."

"Well, what if Dr. Spaw comes out and says you need a mastectomy? I don't want to make that kind of decision without you." His voice was filled with deep concern.

Comforting him, I said gently, "You just know that whatever Dr. Spaw comes out and says that it is from God and you don't worry about it."

The peace I had transcended every fear, every doubt, every worry, every concern. It was a supernatural peace that came from God and His written Word. Isaiah prophetically told us in 53:5, "...the chastisement of our peace is upon him...."

Philippians 6:7 says, "Be anxious for nothing, but in everything by prayer and supplication with thanksgiving, let your requests be made known to God; and the peace of God, which surpasses all understanding, will guard your hearts and minds through Christ Jesus."

What a comfort it was to me to know that these words were written for me! I was fully expecting these truths that had been planted deep inside of me to work. I had a promise from Jesus Himself that says, "It will be done unto you even as you believe."

Just what do you believe? That is what faith boils down to: you, Jesus, and what you believe. Your loved ones aren't responsible for you; your doctors aren't in control. The devil has no say if you've drawn the line and forbid him to cross it. The sickness has no voice— it has to bow to the greater authority of God's Word. It's just you and your Healer. Will you take Him at His Word and believe that what He promised He is able also to perform? If you have fed on His faithfulness and planted the Word in your heart, then the choice is easy. You will have no doubt that the victory He already won belongs to you, too!

He Carried Our Pain

Charlie and I arrived at the Baptist Hospital and began the necessary paperwork before proceeding with the operation. Some might be thinking, *Why did you go ahead with the surgery if you had no doubt that you were healed?*

All I can tell you is that each person has to be led by the Spirit of God for himself or herself about what to do in any given situation. God knows the plans He has for us and I know I had peace about having the surgery. I also know that God did not want me to have any pain in my body and an operation such as this generally had lots of pain associated with it. God was about to demonstrate His mighty power to everyone as the One who bore my sicknesses and carried my pains.

As I waited for the nurse to call me back to be prepped for surgery, I read from *Christ the Healer* by F. F. Bosworth. I knew it was still extremely important to continue to feed my spirit and soul—my mind, will and emotions—with the Word of God and all of His promises to me. You don't fill your "tank" and then let it run dry. You need to refill so that you don't grow slack concerning the truth you have learned. There was no magazine in that waiting room that was more important to me than the Word of God. A magazine wasn't going to do anything for me except steal my Word time. Remember,

Satan comes to steal, kill, and destroy (John 10:10). He wasn't going to give up just because I had made it to the surgery. He's always looking for an opportune time to rob us, and that is all the more reason to stay in the Word. We have to be steadfast and attend to the Word, meditating on it day and night.

Forty-five minutes had passed when they called us back and began to prepare me for surgery. I was donned in a "fashionable" gown, a lovely shower-cap bonnet and all the other bells and whistles. My cheering section: Mother, Peggy, Sister Montell Hardwick, Carol Bryant, and Charlie were all packed in the room with me waiting for the nurses to wheel me to the surgery holding area. Carol began to pray and we all knew that we were trusting the God of Abraham, Isaac, and Jacob for the healing of my body. The same promises God poured out on those three men were available to me through the shed blood of Jesus Christ. Total peace consumed me because I knew these promises were mine. The Scriptures tell us to "hold fast to the profession or confession of our faith without wavering, because He is faithful who promised" (Hebrews 10:23). I knew that I knew the God whom I served was faithful to me.

Through a Door of Faith

The time had finally come. I knew there was no turning back. There was nothing in the past I wanted to return to and nowhere to go but forward—through a door of faith and into the place of trusting God I had been preparing to enter.

I kissed Charlie, said goodbye to my wonderful friends and family, and knew I would never be the same again.

As I waited in the surgery holding area, the anesthesiologist began to administer the anesthesia. Dr. Spaw poked his head in to say hello and to let me know that it was time. I remember being wheeled into the surgery area and then nothing else—I was completely in the hands of my God.

Sometime later, I awoke to the sound of my name, "Deborah…Deborah, wake up. Breathe. That's right, breathe." Shortly after, I was taken to my room to regain full consciousness. I was at the Baptist Hospital as an outpatient, which meant I needed to go home the same day. Charlie was right there by my side. He shared with me how Sister Hardwick had gone back to the church and told everyone there that I had the peace of God all over me. I, too, could sense His peace upon me, but it blessed me to know that believing and receiving the promises of God could also be seen by others.

Bearing Glorious Fruit

I want to make clear that God did not give me this disease, nor did He want me to have it so that He could receive any glory. This belief is another tradition we have been fed, but it bears no truth. God does not receive glory from His children being sick. Yes, I know Matthew 15:30–31 says people gave glory to God when they saw the lame walk and the blind see. People glorified the God of Israel when they saw His power in manifestation. But Jesus said the Father is glorified when we bear much fruit (John 15:8).

Cancer is not fruit, arthritis is not fruit, heart disease and diabetes are not fruits.

Sickness and disease come from the enemy, and what the enemy meant for us is now null and void because Jesus cancelled every debt. He took our place as the final sacrifice, the great Lamb of God who takes away the sins *and sicknesses* of the world. He bought us back from the enemy's grasp and all we would have suffered at Satan's hand. We are God's prized possession, purchased with the life-giving blood of Jesus Christ! Apart from Him we can do nothing, and so the Bible tells us we must abide in Him if we want to bear fruit. Abiding in Him is attending to His Word and doing as He says. It is building a relationship through fellowship with the God of the Universe, our heavenly Father.

Doing Battle With the Bible

God told us that if we would seek Him first, all of the other things we desire would be added to us (Matthew 6:33). The more we know God and His nature, the more keenly aware we become of Satan's schemes. We are then better equipped to respond accordingly when he comes knocking at our door trying to deliver one of his deadly and defeating packages. We simply do what the word says in Second Corinthians 10:5, "Casting down arguments and every high thing that exalts itself against the knowledge of God, bringing every thought into captivity to the obedience of Christ."

Resist the devil from the first sign of attack. Don't give him any room by waiting to see what he is planning next. The Bible says he comes for the Word's sake (Mark 4:17). He torments us because he knows he can get away with it, keeping our mind busy with his lies and negative thoughts. Then, before we know it, he has stolen our Word time or our praise time.

The way to battle the enemy is with the Word; the same weapon Jesus used against him in the wilderness where He fasted for forty days and forty nights. The authority Jesus delegated to us in Matthew 28:18 is at our disposal, and Ephesians 6:11 describes the whole amour of God we must put on so that we will be able to stand against the wiles (schemes) of the devil. There is no substitute for time in the Word; it is the only way we will become familiar with the promises of God and how to receive them.

We can know something but not apply it in our lives and never receive the benefits of it. For example, if I put $10,000 in your bank account and you knew it but didn't write any checks against it, that money would do you no good. God's provisional promises are the same way; all of His promises are available to us in abundance if we will simply make a withdrawal and activate them through faith.

Faith Always Rises to the Top

I was blessed to have faithful friends and family visit me immediately after the surgery. Donnie Wood and Joy Wright came to the hospital, along with my children and grandchildren. I sensed so much love as they stood around my bed and talked with me.

Under my right armpit where Dr. Spaw had removed the lymph nodes, a drain tube had been inserted. Tubes from both the IV's and the drain tube were hanging all around me. One of my grandchildren was determined to walk on them and, needless to say, his uncle reprimanded him.

I could see the concern on my children's faces as they stared wide-eyed at all the equipment hooked up to me. I'm sure it brought back memories of how their Pappaw looked and what he had gone through. What they didn't see, however, was the assurance I had in God and His Word. They didn't know or understand these promises because, like many people—Charlie and I included up until this point—they had never been taught God's Word concerning healing.

I have found that living in a natural world, we often look only to natural means to work through problems. We think we can handle whatever comes ourselves, or we look to our doctor to see us through. But we serve a supernatural God who provides supernatural healing beyond what any person or medicine could do! He is willing and able to perform His Word if only we will call on Him and put our trust in His promises.

71

I appreciate medical science and what doctors can do, and in no way am I being critical of doctors. I know many doctors practicing medicine who believe in and trust God, Dr. Spaw included. My point is, don't limit your help to a doctor, when the Great Physician is standing by ready to restore you to perfect health!

After all the visitors had gone and the excitement had died down, one of the first things I noticed was my veracious appetite. I called for the nurse to ask if I could have something to eat. "Honey, you are on a clear liquid diet, I'm sorry, but you can't have anything to eat."

Liquid just wasn't going to cut it, not with my appetite. "But I'm really hungry," I insisted. Their policy after surgery is no solid food because most likely it's all going to come up. It's quite common to be nauseated to the point of vomiting following anesthesia and surgery. I knew this to be true based on my experience in the Sam's parking lot following the first surgery. I must have looked so pitiful to the nurse that she finally gave in to my plea for food. "I have some Jell-O cups," she suggested, "would you like one?" I jumped at the chance. She brought it and I think I inhaled it in all of ten seconds.

"I am still hungry," I told her.

"Would you like another one?" she asked.

What do you suppose my answer was? "Yes!" I ate that one too, and asked for more. She was trying her best to talk me out of eating anything else to spare me from what she was accustomed to seeing. The last thing patients need after major surgery is to be nauseated and vomiting. But you see, I never professed that I was sick. You can't believe for your healing and then tell everyone how sick you are. I was doing just as the Scriptures say in James 1:6–8: "But let him ask in faith, with no doubting, for he who doubts is like a wave of the sea driven and tossed by the wind. For let not that man suppose that he will receive anything from the Lord; he is a double-minded man, unstable in all his ways."

If you are being tossed to and fro like waves of the sea, check and see if perhaps you are believing one thing and saying another. Sometimes we are not even aware that what we say is contrary to what we have prayed. Often people's questions cause us to feel obligated to answer a certain way that may not be in line with the Word. We have to be grounded in the Word to the point we will not waiver. Just as water and oil don't mix, neither do faith and doubt; one always rises to the top. I was determined that faith was rising to the top for me.

We Have What we Say

I looked at the nurse one more time with such pity for myself and once again voiced my hunger. "I have half a turkey sandwich," she said, "would you like to have it?"

"Yes!" I told her. (I was hoping for something a little more substantial than Jell-O.) I ate it in only a few bites. I know what many people are thinking right about now: *She's going to be sick!* After the sandwich, I was offered a bowl of noodle soup, and yes, I ate that too. By this time I finally felt satisfied. I also had to use the restroom.

73

With all of her running back and forth to get me food, the nurse failed to give me instructions about the drain tube, so when I got out of bed to use the restroom, the drain tube bag was dangling from my arm. "What's this?" I asked, surprised.

The nurse explained to me what it was and pinned it to my gown, out of the way. I used the restroom without assistance and crawled back into bed. Just then, Charlie came back to my room and sat down beside me. We decided that it would be best if I spent the night there at the hospital so they could monitor my progress. We knew some of the grandchildren and kids were staying at our house, and thought it would be a good idea for us to get a good nights rest at the hospital.

We called for the nurse and told her of our plans. She went to work making the necessary arrangements to transport me to another part of the hospital for overnight patients. As soon as she finished the paperwork, off we went. For Charlie and me, our night at the hospital was like a night of vacation.

Once we were settled in our room, I suggested that Charlie go to the cafeteria and get something to eat. He went, only to find that it was already closed. The time was 8:00 P.M. and we were both getting tired. There was a drive-through place just near the hospital, but Charlie was hesitant to leave me alone in case I needed anything. I assured him that I would be surrounded with God's angels and that no plague or calamity would come near my dwelling (Psalm 91:10). After all, this hospital room was my dwelling place, at least for overnight.

When Charlie returned, oh what a treat I had in store! He brought back two pints of cookies and cream ice cream, one for him and one for me. I sat up in bed and ate the whole thing! When the nurse came in to give me the pain medicine for the night, I told him that I had no pain, but I would take it and have a good night's rest. I took the medicine, kissed Charlie, and drifted off to sleep.

No, I didn't wake up sick in the middle of the night because of all I had eaten. In fact, I had a peaceful and restful night, and awoke in the morning hungrier than ever. A breakfast tray arrived in my room with eggs, bacon, coffee and toast, and I ate every bite. Now I was simply waiting to be discharged and sent home. I needed to get home because the conference was starting the next day, and I had eight guests arriving from Canada to stay in our home. When they learned of the surgery I was to have, they offered not to come, or to arrange for other accommodations, but I wouldn't hear of it. I didn't know any of them, but I knew they and their church had been praying for me. The daughter of one of the individuals had stayed with us once while attending a YWAM function, and that was our connection to this group. I was really looking forward to meeting them, and felt honored that they would be staying with us.

The time came for me to be released from the hospital. I thanked the staff for their kind service, and Charlie and I headed home, full of joy and expectancy for all that lay ahead. It was 11:00 A.M. when we arrived at home. Charlie helped to tuck me into bed. My precious grandchildren gathered around me and we visited for a while about their adventures and mine. Then they all piled in the car and headed home to Alabama.

My Mother came to stay with us and to help in any way she could. I knew deep down she must have been so concerned for her "baby girl." She was so protective of me, not wanting me to do anything, lest I strain myself. One thing I had to do was have my hair fixed before church Sunday. I had fifty-two tables to set for breakfast for Monday morning's conference, and volunteers would be waiting on me. I certainly didn't want to go to church with "bed hair." My hair looked like it had been separated by a strong wind, the entire back looked just as flat as a board.

I encouraged Mother to take me over to my sister Peggy's beauty salon to have my hair styled. She drove ever so slowly all the way there, trying not to hit any bumps along the way. When we arrived, no one could believe I was up and around, let alone at the beauty salon. *Who would care about having their hair done at a time like this?* they wondered. I can't stress enough, you can't claim to believe for healing and then talk about being sick and feeling bad. I am not saying that when you're in faith for healing that you don't have pain. What I am saying is that you don't have to give the devil place in your life by agreeing with the symptoms he's trying to heap on you. The Scriptures plainly tell us that whatever comes out of our mouth is what we will have. Have you ever felt a symptom come and then the more you talked about it the worse you felt? You gave that sickness place with your words. You can talk yourself into almost anything.

Instead of confessing the problem, claim the answer: "By the stripes of Jesus, I am healed!"

A Confirming Dream

After I had my hair styled, Mother and I went home. In about an hour, the first group of guests arrived. We showed them to the rooms they would be sleeping in and gave them some time to get settled. Then we all gathered around the kitchen table. They began to share with us how their church had been praying for me and how grateful they were that under the circumstances we had still allowed them to stay in our home. At the time, none of us had a clue what a blessing this group would actually be to us. God, in His infinite wisdom, had again seen ahead and provided. It is wonderful to meet God's children from other places of the world.

As we continued to fellowship, the second group arrived. We got them settled and then once again gathered around the kitchen table. One of the young men present began to talk to me directly. His name was David. He was a rather shy young man, which confirmed God's power on him as he boldly shared what he had seen. He began to relay to me a dream he had. "Deborah, I don't know you right? I have never seen you before have I?

"That's right, David. You don't know me and have never seen me before, not even in a picture," I told him.

He shared with me that in his dream, he had seen me and he saw Jesus standing over me healing my body of this breast cancer.

I believed what this young man saw in his dream was true. His dream confirmed what I already believed to be true; Jesus had healed me! When we believe without doubt, God is able to perform His Word in our lives. Isaiah 55:11 tells us that His Word will not return to Him void, but will accomplish that which pleases Him. It pleases Him that we, His children, be well.

God also told us that He sent His Word and healed us, and delivered us from our destruction (Psalm 107:20). I knew without a doubt that He had done this for me. My faith in the Word had activated its power in my life. Healing didn't just come automatically, it took a lot of time and effort to plant the Word on healing in my heart to the point that my faith in God and His Word eliminated any doubt.

We visited into the evening then said our good nights. We wanted to be sure that everyone had adequate rest before the four days of meetings started. The next morning our guests awoke and excitedly began getting ready for church. I had decided to go after the service to meet with the volunteers and make sure the dining room was ready for breakfast the following morning. My sister Peggy came by the house and picked Mother and me up to take us to the church. When we arrived, I found my volunteers there busily attending to their assigned tasks. I had just stepped into the dining room when Pastor Hardwick saw me and made a beeline over to me. "What are you doing here, Deborah?" he asked.

I remember telling him, "Pastor, I have things to do. And besides all that, you don't pray for a healing and go around claiming to be sick."

The look on his face said, "Girl, considering the circumstances you should be home in bed!"

I promised him it would only be a short visit and I'd go straight home. After thanking the volunteers for their faithfulness to the Lord we did just that. We had a wonderful time of fellowship with our guests that afternoon, then caught a nap before the evening service.

God's Power Revealed

Mother and I stayed home that evening. I wanted to be fresh for our 325 guests scheduled for breakfast the next morning. Once again, when I arrived at the church the next day, all of my volunteers were in place and ready to go to work. Mother and Peggy helped too and were an added blessing.

Breakfast came off flawlessly, and then it was time to prepare for lunch. We reset all the tables making sure every last thing was in place. Approximately 315 were expected for lunch, and as we waited, I went around the corner to the church offices to call Dr. Spaw as he instructed me to do on Monday. He wasn't available, so I left my pager number. When I came back to join the others, Alfred McCroskey, one of our church missionaries, met me at the beverage table. He told me that Charlie needed me to come upstairs to the registration table. "Alfred," I told him, "if Charlie wants me he's going to have to come to me; I've got 315 people to attend to at the moment."

Mother and Peggy were standing to the right of me, just as they were in my dream. Just then, I felt someone put both their hands on my shoulders. I turned around to face Charlie. I will never forget his words. "Deborah, Dr. Spaw just called. He said the cancer is all gone! They didn't find a trace of cancer, not even in the fourteen lymph nodes that they removed."

The scene was one of exuberant joy and celebration. We all began to praise the Lord simultaneously. Those who knew I had been diagnosed with breast cancer lifted their hands toward heaven and worshipped the Lord. Mother and Peggy were hugging me and crying, so thankful to God for His mighty work.

The rest of the day was filled with rejoicing. No words can describe how we felt as we basked in the glory of the fulfillment of God's promises. Charlie and I had always believed I was healed, and had experienced God's blessings great and small all along the way. Now, everyone else had seen the mighty hand of God on my life. Brother Jim's prophecy was coming to pass: God was showing me His great power. I would now be a witness of this same power, telling everyone that they, too, could experience the healing power of God. The power of the Word is available to all who will learn God's promises and stand on them.

That evening after the service I found my friend Gail. If you recall, she is the nurse who explained things to me over the phone the same night I was diagnosed. I had asked her to look at the bandage that was over the drain tube. We stepped into one of the classrooms, closed the door, and she took a look. "We really need to change this dressing," she said, so we sent Charlie to the store to buy some gauze bandages and tape. When he returned, Gail carefully redressed the area over the drain tube. "Be sure to save some of the pain medication," Gail told me. "You're going to need it when Dr. Spaw removes the drain tube; that is always very painful."

The conference continued for two more days and was wonderful. It was always such a let down when conferences ended. All of our guests returned home and the buzz in our house was gone. Wednesday night Pastor Hardwick held a pastor's reception in his office, and at that time shared with all the ministers how God had healed me of breast cancer. They, too, broke into spontaneous worship when they heard the testimony. It is one thing to hear about someone being healed, it is another to actually see someone be healed. We walk by faith and not by sight, but God uses demonstrations of His power to help the "unbelieving" believe. For some people "seeing is believing" as the familiar expression says.

Pastor Hardwick also reported to the congregation in a church service about God healing me. I had the opportunity to share with "many people" as well about the Lord's healing power just as God said I would.

Never Alone

Two weeks had passed and I had an office visit scheduled with Dr. Spaw on May 2. Charlie had gone with me for every visit I had to Dr. Spaw's office—until today. This particular day Charlie couldn't go. I told him not to feel bad; I could drive myself. It was not a big deal because I was just certain Dr. Spaw wouldn't take the drain tube out today: it was still draining 30 cc's of liquid, and that was way too much for the tube to come out.

When I was taken into the examination room however, it looked like a surgical unit and I knew I was in trouble. No Charlie and no pain medication! As I lay down on the examination table, I prayed, "Lord, don't let Dr. Spaw do anything against Your will for me. Let every word that comes out of his mouth be from You." I knew that if Satan had a chance, he would use the removal of this drain tube against me.

Dr. Spaw greeted me with a familiar smile, then proceeded to tell me that today he would be removing the drain tube from under my arm area. When I questioned him about it, he said it had been two weeks and it was time for the tube to come out. Though Charlie wasn't with me, the God who healed me was, and He would see me through this procedure. I quietly meditated on the fact that I didn't need pain medication because Jesus bore my pain. I didn't need Charlie because I had Jesus with me. My faithful Father had never left me alone.

I can't say I necessarily "felt" strong, but by faith I said, "I can do all things through Christ who strengthens me." I turned my head away as Dr. Spaw began the procedure, and confessed over and over, "Jesus bore my pain. Jesus bore my pain. Jesus bore my pain." I could hear Dr. Spaw moving around, so I turned to him and asked, "Are you finished?"

To my surprise, he was! "Yes," he said. "See?" He was holding a tube at least five inches long. I never felt a thing! God is so good and His mercies endure forever. He always honors His Word. Jesus not only bore the sickness and disease that had attacked my body, He also bore my pains and sorrow (Isaiah 53:4).

Claim the promises of God for whatever condition might be plaguing you. Is it a blood disease, bone ailment, or hearing impairment? Perhaps you've lost function in your body due to a traumatic accident. No case is too difficult or specialized for the Great Physician. Become familiar with what the Word says concerning healing. Study God's promises, making them your own. Hearing the Word, meditating in scriptures that are alive with healing power, then believing and speaking God's promises will change whatever it is that has affected your body or mind. Yes, it takes time. We must be steadfast in the Word, attending to it day and night.

When God's Word gets in your heart, it will come out of your mouth and His promises will be fulfilled in your life. I am no different from you. The Word says God is no respecter of persons. What He did for me, He will do for anyone—anyone who will believe.

Chapter 6

All Worth it for One

The road of faith Charlie and I had been traveling opened up a completely new world to us. It was a world of possibility and promise, not just for us to discover, but also for those we would encounter along the way. What we were learning would soon permeate a place where few, if any, physical healings were seen—the radiation center.

Yes, I knew I was healed through faith in God's Word; Dr. Spaw saw the results and believed the same as we did. We also all knew it seemed right to follow through with the scheduled radiation treatments. I remember praying about the treatments and telling the Lord, "If I could share what You have done for me with just one person at this center, it will all be worth it."

I knew the dangers associated with radiation therapy. My Daddy had undergone treatments from the same oncologist to whom Dr.

Spaw had referred me. Each time Daddy went for a treatment, He came home feeling worse than he did before he left the house. His skin where they directed the treatments became hard and burned, and he had markings all over the area where the radiation was administered.

On occasion, I was the one who took Daddy to his appointments. Vividly etched in my memory was the atmosphere at the center and the look on everyone's faces. It was always dark and depressing there. Everyone looked half-dead; they were lifeless and void of hope. The spirits of sickness, disease, pain, dread, depression, fear and death pervaded every room. It certainly was no place to "hang out." I knew if Satan could, he would use the memory of Daddy's treatments against me. I stood firm on the truth that the life of God was in me; Jesus came that I might have life and have it more abundantly!

My first visit to Dr. Lloyd, the radiation oncologist, was on June 3. Several of the staff recognized me from when I had brought Daddy in just one year earlier. They were saddened that now I was their patient. What a surprise they were in for with me and Christ my Healer!

As I waited in the examination room for Dr. Lloyd, I closed my eyes and pictured slipping my hand into God's. "You've taken me this far," I told Him. "I trust you to take me all the way through." Just then, Dr. Lloyd stepped into the room. He was a tall, thin man. The deep lines in his face suggested that he was carrying a heavy load.

How could he not be, surrounded by death most of the time? Most of the people he saw at this stage did not outlive the disease.

As we went through a polite introduction, I looked at him and asked, "Dr. Lloyd, are you a Christian?"

A surprised grin softened the lines in his face: "Why, Yes Deborah, I am," he responded.

"Dr. Lloyd, you know that God has healed me and I am only here because Dr. Spaw made me come. It was part of the deal I made with him so that I wouldn't have to have a mastectomy."

"Yes, I know all about that Deborah. But we all need all the help we can get."

Little did he know the miracle he would soon witness—God's mighty power demonstrated for all to see!

Dr. Lloyd proceeded to explain the details of how I needed to be marked for the treatments. In one sense, it reminded me of the mark of the beast! And that is exactly what this mark was like, a mark of despair, a mark one could not get rid of, a sign marking "the end." For many, these marks were the end.

I was led across the hall to a dark room where I had to lie on a cold, hard table waiting for the procedure to begin. I recall the day Daddy went for his markings. They left him on the table for some time and he was very uncomfortable. When the technician finally came back into the room, he asked her if she had enjoyed her lunch. "Mr. Malone," she told him, "I haven't been to lunch."

"Well, you've been gone long enough to have had lunch!" he charged. I don't know what went through the technician's mind at that moment, but I do know they all grew to love Daddy.

I had to admit as I lay on the table replaying this scene that Daddy was right. It seemed like the technicians just left you there and disappeared. *Where did they go anyway?* I wondered.

Dwelling in the Secret Place

Finally, someone returned to my room and began the marking. I left the room with green X's all over my right breast, which remained there until the last treatment was given. I entered this phase of the treatment fully aware of radiation's effects. *And you still decided to go through with it?* some might be asking. God gave me the promise of Psalm 91:1–16 in His Word:

> **He that dwelleth in the secret place of the most High shall abide under the shadow of the Almighty.**
>
> **I will say of the Lord, He is my refuge and my fortress: my God; in him will I trust.**
>
> **Surely he shall deliver thee from the snare of the fowler, and from the noisome pestilence.**
>
> **He shall cover thee with his feathers, and under his wings shalt thou trust: his truth shall be thy shield and buckler.**

Thou shalt not be afraid for the terror by night; nor for the arrow that flieth by day;

Nor for the pestilence that walketh in darkness; nor for the destruction that wasteth at noonday.

A thousand shall fall at thy side, and ten thousand at thy right hand; but it shall not come nigh thee.

Only with thine eyes shalt thou behold and see the reward of the wicked.

Because thou hast made the Lord, which is my refuge, even the most High, thy habitation;

There shall no evil befall thee, neither shall any plague come nigh thy dwelling.

For he shall give his angels charge over thee, to keep thee in all thy ways.

They shall bear thee up in their hands, lest thou dash thy foot against a stone.

Thou shalt tread upon the lion and adder: the young lion and the dragon shalt thou trample under feet.

Because he hath set his love upon me, therefore will I deliver him: I will set him on high, because he hath known my name.

He shall call upon me, and I will answer him: I will be with him in trouble; I will deliver him, and honour him.

With long life will I satisfy him, and shew him my salvation.

All of God's provision for divine protection is contingent upon us dwelling in the "secret place"—giving Him first place in our lives. We will come to know God through His Word and through times of intimate fellowship with Him. We cannot have confidence in His promises unless we've studied them and know what they entail. Then, once we've become familiar with God's promises, we must remain steadfast in the Word. Being steadfast means to be firm, secure, and to dwell in and inhabit. Your home is your abode or dwelling place. How much time do you spend in your home? It takes time to dwell. Dwelling is more than speaking a quick confession here or there when we have a need. To dwell means to stay in God and in His Word day and night, allowing it to sink into our heart until it comes out of our mouth and begins to govern our life.

Each day before I left for treatment, I positioned the angels to stand at every entrance and every exit to the hospital. I prayed that God would grant wisdom and knowledge to everyone on staff who would be working with me directly. I prayed and spoke the Word of God from the time I left my home until I walked back out of the building. I had a desire in my heart to share the eternal hope of Christ with the other patients there.

Each day, the routine was the same. The appointment began in the women's area, where I changed into a lovely hospital gown. Thankfully, it was the kind that tied in the front, making it so much more modest. Then I filed to the waiting area and sat waiting with all the other patients. Most of the faces were filled with fear. Their heads hung low as they spoke of either how badly they felt or about how many treatments they had remaining. Many rummaged through the supply of magazines tattered with use, and thumbed through the pages while waiting. There is nothing wrong with looking at magazines, but waiting for radiation at a hospital was neither the time nor the place.

It was so sad to watch desperate people remain helpless and hopeless with not a clue as to what to do. Just as I needed to, these people needed to know how to get into the Word and apply it to their individual situations. I tried to share what God had done for me with as many as I could. Sadly, most of them looked at me as if I had that third eyeball. The Bible says, "My people are destroyed for lack of knowledge," and that is exactly what was happening to these precious people. Satan, the thief, was stealing, killing, and destroying their bodies and their lives.

There was no way I was going to allow the devil to harm my body while I was undergoing radiation treatments. I know that he meant it all for my harm, but the God that I serve takes whatever the enemy means for harm and makes good out of it.

Name it and Claim it!

I will never grow tired of declaring the promises of God, because faith comes by hearing and hearing. Learn the Word of God. Speak it out of your mouth. Let Satan know that "Greater is he that is in you, than he that is in the world." You don't have to be afraid of sickness and disease. Don't cower in its presence; it has to bow in yours, because the Greater One lives and dwells in you!

Trust in Jesus as Savior, Lord, and Healer. Learn to depend upon Him. Don't let what He has provided for you go unclaimed. Yes, name it and claim it! Tell Satan he is not going to make you sick and he is not going to put fear on you. He cannot do anything to you except for what you allow him to do. You have been given power and authority to trample on serpents and scorpions and over all the power of the enemy (Luke 10:19). You have access to the same power Jesus walked in while He was on the earth. You need only to learn to use this power.

Satan is not afraid of you and what you can do to him, but he is afraid of what you can do with God's Word. The authority of the Word is the enemy's doom. The Bible says the devil is under our feet because as Christians our position is in Christ, seated with Jesus in heavenly places. That's a good place from which to kick the devil in the teeth! Remember who you are and remember *Who's* you are, and don't let the enemy talk you out of the promises of God!

Divine Protection

It was the third day of the treatment, and as I waited for my turn, I prayed specifically for God's protection from the equipment that administered the radiation. I also asked for wisdom and knowledge for the technicians who would be operating the equipment.

Finally, I was called for the treatment. I lay on the table and waited as the technician prepared the equipment. She turned the machine so that it would beam the radiation toward the outside of my right breast. Then she left the room while the machine began to operate. I had always counted to see how long each administration was going to last. It had generally been taking twenty-five seconds. This time, however, the technician was not coming back into the room to turn the machine to administer radiation to the left side.

I stayed calm and continued to pray for God to give her wisdom and knowledge. I knew something was not right. In a few moments she returned with Brenda, the technician who had treated Daddy. They walked behind the head of the table to the huge machine that administered the radiation. I couldn't turn around to see what was happening because the markings were lined up directly where the laser beams needed to go, and I was given strict instructions to lie very still throughout the entire treatment. "You must always make sure this is down," Brenda instructed, as she clamped something into position behind me.

93

That very moment I knew why God had led me to pray so specifically that morning. He had protected me just as I had asked Him to and just as He had promised in His Word.

The Sword of the Spirit

God has given us all the ammunition we need to overcome the enemy, but most of us have the "Barney Fife Syndrome;" we have a gun but no bullets!

Load your spirit with a supply of Word ammunition and speak that Word every chance you get. Before long you'll be able to aim, shoot, and hit your target dead-center every time!

Day after day, I continued to pray before and during each radiation treatment. I never failed to pray for protection. I knew Satan would try to kill me if he had half a chance, and I certainly wasn't going to give it to him. I used the sword of the Spirit—the Word of God—which is sharper than any two-edged sword. I continually confessed God's healing promises because it wouldn't have done me any good to leave the "sword" in its sheath; I had to speak God's Word out of my mouth.

With every passing day I built relationships with all the women working at the treatment center. They were all so nice to me. They remembered my Daddy very well, and talked to me often about his and my Mother's restaurants. They told me about all the recipes he had shared with them and of the stories he had told them about his life.

As I walked through the memory of his visits in my mind, I made a stark contrast between his course and mine. When Daddy was diagnosed, we didn't know what God had promised in His Word; and therefore, Satan had stolen Daddy's life from him through ignorance of the Word.

I could also look around me at the other patients and see the enemy's work. One woman had gotten blisters all under her arm and over her entire breast. Another patient experienced a machine's malfunction and received two treatments at once. Of course no one on staff told us this, but the patients shared their experiences in confidence.

I could tangibly see God's promises of protection shielding me from every weapon the enemy tried to form against me, not one of his schemes could prosper.

Divine Visitation

June 27 will forever be embedded in my memory. It was the eighteenth day of the treatments, and I was lying on the table waiting for radiation to be administered to the right side of my breast. The technician had positioned the equipment, then left the room.

As I began to count off the seconds before her return, the most awesome presence filled the room. Out of the corner of my eye, I could see a tall shape hovering to my right shoulder about six feet or so from the table. I couldn't turn to look at it directly because I was already in position for the laser beams.

Words cannot describe the glorious feeling I experienced; it was magnificent, awesome, and exciting all at the same time. I didn't want this feeling to end. I found myself saying, "Lord, is that You?" It only could have been Him for me to have such jubilance, peace and complete trust.

I didn't hear a voice, but in an instant I had a knowing inside of me that He was present in the room with me. I knew His Word was truth and that He would protect me in all my ways. Only a glimpse of His glory brought so much life to me. To know that we will spend eternity with Him basking and worshipping in His presence forever and ever is such a blessed promise.

As soon as I arrived at home, I ran to find Charlie to tell him what had happened. My words came pouring out like a flood—the same presence saturating me all over again as I relayed to him my experience.

Charlie's response was so matter-of-fact: "You pray for God's protection from the time you leave the house until the time you return. I guess the Lord decided to show you that He was doing just that," he said, as he smiled in confirming belief.

The truth is, my relationship with the Lord had grown so close as I spent time with Him in prayer and through His Word that I wasn't entirely surprised that He visited me, though I was remarkably honored. I had never experienced His awesomeness quite this way before. This was a first as was the dream He had given me at the beginning of this journey. Life with God is truly an adventure!

Divine Appointment

Every opportunity I could find, I witnessed the goodness of God to people during the treatments. The beginning of one such opportunity presented itself on July 10, the twenty-fifth day of treatment. I had been sent across the hall for the markings of the boosters. At this stage they remarked my breast in order to administer a much more intense dose of radiation.

Louise, the woman who would be administering the radiation, and Dr. Lloyd were both examining my right breast tissue. Dr. Lloyd was amazed. "Deborah, your skin looks so good that I am going to start the boosters tomorrow. Normally we wait about two weeks, but with your skin looking so good that won't be necessary."

I could look around me at the other patients and see the difference between my skin and theirs. I knew that God had preserved and protected me. Even my sister Peggy asked me one day, "What are you doing, your skin looks so good?"

"I think it's called radiation," I teased, "Don't I just glow?!"

I knew from the first day I met Louise that God was working in her heart. She had that "look," as if she knew there was more to life than what she was experiencing. July 16, the twenty-ninth day of treatment, Louise asked me, "Deborah, how do you women get through this? I get up some days and can't make my hair do what it's supposed to and I think *I* have a problem. Then I get to work and see all of you ladies dealing with a life and death disease…how do you manage?"

It was as if I could hear the angels of heaven rejoicing, knowing that I had an open door to tell this woman of my wonderful Lord. I smiled and remembered the words I had spoken to God: "If I can share with just one person, Lord, it will all be worth taking these treatments." *Yes, Lord, she's the one!* I thought.

I looked her right in the eyes and said, "Louise, I don't know how the other ladies get through this, but I can tell you how I do." And then I began to share Jesus with her. I told her how He died for me on the cross and bore not only all my sins, but also all the sickness, disease and pain I might ever experience. I just let the words flow straight from my heart to hers.

After the treatment was finished, I was walking down the hall to leave when I came across Sister Dotie Osteen's book: *Healed of Cancer* along with healing scripture cards in the racks where they kept all the patient information about radiation and chemotherapy. My insides filled with emotion as I lifted the book off the rack and started back down the hall to find Louise. I knew this was a divine appointment. I handed her the book and told her, "Louise, you read this book and see how the God whom I serve heals His children. He is ever-faithful to perform His Word." She took the book in her hands and offered a hopeful smile, as if she knew too that someone had orchestrated this moment.

The Fourth Man in the Fire

July 19, the last day, treatment number thirty-two. I came equipped with a small pocket book presenting the plan of salvation in the back and gave it to Louise. She was so amazed that I would be interested in her enough to remember her concern. I knew that she was searching. Her eyes and words all pointed to a hungry heart. She saw patients every day in various stages of disease, most of them had no hope. Now, she had seen with her very own eyes that Jesus was my Healer, and death and decay did not have to be the outcome for anyone. Yes, there are wonderful doctors too—I had the best—but we can't put our trust in doctors for healing. The only One we can depend upon for total deliverance from anything this world can inflict is Christ the Healer.

He had delivered me from every evil thing while undergoing these treatments. I was never sick, though I was told to expect it. I was never tired, though they told me it was inevitable. As a matter of fact, I never missed a day of work! My skin looked so wonderful Dr. Lloyd told me if he hadn't known I had been there, he wouldn't have known I had been there!

This was all a testimony of our faithful Father God. The whole experience reminded me of the three Hebrew children—Shadrach, Meshach, and Abednego—in the third chapter of Daniel. They were put in a fiery furnace on order of the king because they refused to worship the golden image that the king had constructed. The fire was made seven times hotter than usual as a result of the king's fury of their defiance. The fire was so hot that it killed the king's men who were assigned to throw the Hebrew children in the furnace.

As Shadrach, Meshach, and Abednego fell down, bound in the fire, the king noticed a fourth person in the fire with them. "Did we not cast three men bound into the midst of the fire?" King Nebuchadnezzer asked in verse 24.

"True, O king," his men responded.

"...I see four men loose, walking in the midst of the fire, and they have no hurt; and the form of the fourth is like the Son of God."

The king called for them to come out from the midst of the fire. "And the princes, governors, and captains, and the king's counsellers, being gathered together, saw these men, upon whose bodies the fire had no power, nor was an hair of their head singed, neither were their coats changed, nor the smell of fire had passed on them," (Daniel :27).

Truly, "the fourth man in the fire" had delivered me from radiation's destruction just as He had delivered the three Hebrew children from the fiery furnace. He is the same yesterday, today, and forever!

Dealt Another Blow

Although the thirty-two treatments were over, the visits to the doctor were not. Following the radiation, I was scheduled to see Dr. Hannah, an orthopedic surgeon. At one point in the treatment, my rotator cuff was pulled from it's place in the socket. No, the devil couldn't get to me through the equipment or effects of the radiation, so he threw me a curve ball.

We must understand that just because a person is a believer does not mean he or she is exempt from the attacks of the enemy. In fact, it is often the contrary; believers—especially those who know the Word—can become a target for the enemy. Attacks do not indicate that a person is not in faith or that he or she has some hidden sin. Attacks come simply because we are human. Don't be condemned if it seems one thing after another is coming against you. Psalm 34:19 says, "Many are the afflictions of the righteous: but the Lord delivereth him out of them *all*."

I had been doing everything I knew to do to activate God's protection, but one day when I was lying on the examination table receiving treatments, the technician tried to adjust my position by pulling on my gown. Instead, she placed her hand around my shoulder, and when she pulled, my shoulder was dislocated. It hurt, but thinking it was just sore, I never said anything.

Day after day, it became increasingly difficult to put my hand behind my head and keep my elbow on the table, which I needed to do for the treatments. When Dr. Lloyd observed my inability to keep my arm in the correct position, he asked me what happened and I had to explain the unfortunate accident this technician had made. He then sent me to Dr. Hannah for x-rays of my rotator cuff.

Satan is not very smart. He should have known by now that I was standing on God's healing promises and that He would somehow make this situation turn out for my good. It made no difference to me if the healing was for an infected gum, breast cancer, or a damaged shoulder; the same healing promises apply to any sickness, disease, or accident the enemy brings.

After Dr. Hannah examined my shoulder, he advised me to begin physical therapy at once. "If the shoulder doesn't heal itself through therapy," he told me "then I will need to do surgery." He would perform what they call "manipulation" in medical terms. The description alone sounded horrible. The patient is put under anesthesia and the doctor twists the affected arm 360 degrees. That was all I needed to hear. "God healed me of breast cancer, Dr. Hannah, and if He can do that, He can take care of a frozen shoulder," I told him.

I knew Dr. Hannah was a Christian, so I asked him if he would agree with me for healing. "Of course I will Deborah, but you have to do your part too," he said.

"Agreed!" I told him, and headed downstairs to meet the therapist. Amazingly, the therapist was one of my Christian friends from Christ Church! God is so good! Again, He had orchestrated this meeting down to the last detail. I shared with Brent, the therapist, that I was believing God would heal my shoulder, and that surgery would not be necessary. I then asked if he would agree with me for my healing. "Yes, Deborah, I will agree with you in faith, but you will need to follow my instructions carefully." I told him that wouldn't be a problem; I had gotten pretty good at following instructions. That is just what I was doing with God's Word: attending to it, keeping it before my eyes, putting it into my ears, and speaking it out of my mouth. Instructions I could do!

Stand Your Ground

As Brent prepared the paperwork, I took a moment to reflect on all that was happening. I knew Satan would have loved for me to have to go through more surgery, trying to wear me down and discourage my faith. But this only fueled my faith! Now I would have more opportunities to testify of God's healing power and tell of His goodness to even more people. It doesn't matter what Satan tries to "dish out," we don't have to take what Jesus already took! Get serious about what Jesus bought and paid for with His own precious blood, and don't let the enemy steal it. He'll try to steal the Word in your heart, the joy in your spirit, the peace in your mind, and the health in your body. Develop a conquering spirit. Stand your ground with your feet planted firmly on the rock, and *nothing* will be able to shake your foundation.

Stay on guard at all times. When symptoms come don't say, "I think I'm coming down with the flu and won't be able to go to work," say, "No, devil, you take your symptoms and go! My body is the temple of the Holy Spirit and I didn't order what you're serving. I am not under the curse of the law, I live under the law of the Spirit of life in Christ Jesus!"

Be Tenacious not Complacent

Unfortunately, most of us are spiritually lazy and don't ward the enemy off at the first sign of his attack. Instead, we think about how we *feel* and even begin to say how we feel rather than taking the time to speak the promises of God. Diligently attending to God's Word takes time and effort on our part. We can't be complacent about God's promises, we have to be tenacious about them! The armor of God's Word is our cover, shielding us from the enemy's schemes. When we are full of God's Word we will be able to replace lies with truth, weakness with strength, worry with peace, grumbling with praise, doubt with hope, and fear with faith!

We can't wait until we are in six feet of water to learn how to swim. That is what happened to me, and it was no one's fault but my own. It's up to each one of us to learn God's promises of healing and prosperity from the Bible and then begin to apply them to our lives. Once we know them, we can share them with others, giving them hope and a future. There are so many hurting people searching for answers. You could be the very one to bring them the light! How will they know unless you go and tell them? God has made provision for everyone to walk in His promises and we must be ready in season and out of season to give an account of what we have seen and heard. That is what it means to be a witness. If we are going to live as more than conquerors in this world, then we have to know the authority Jesus delegated to us through His name and His Word. And, we must be proficient in using it!

Resist Steadfast in the Faith

No matter how far you go in God, don't be surprised to find Satan right there waiting to deal you another blow. He will never give up. First Peter 5:8 says, "Be sober, be vigilant; because your adversary the devil, as a roaring lion, walketh about, seeking whom he may devour."

Notice the Bible doesn't say the devil *is* a roaring lion, it says he walks about *as* a roaring lion. He is all bark and no bite! He'll talk long enough to get us to listen to him, trying to convince us that we are sick, broke, or will never amount to anything. He is the accuser of the brethren, and the way we combat his lies is to do as verse 9 says: "Whom resist stedfast in the faith, knowing that the same afflictions are accomplished in your brethren that are in the world."

How do we resist steadfast in the faith? We study the Scriptures and then mix faith with what we have heard. Hebrews 4:2 says that the word was given to God's people for their good, but didn't profit them because they didn't mix faith with it. How does faith come? According to Romans 10:17, "Faith comes by hearing and hearing by the word of God." That's why I am being repetitious, writing over and over to you what I learned from the Word. I want faith to be built in your heart until you believe and are saturated with this truth!

Deborah M. West

Speak the Promises

I went to therapy twice a week for a total of two months. During my sessions, Brent introduced me to a dear woman who had already had two manipulations and extended therapy and still wasn't able to raise her arm as high as I could after I had been there for only one week. Granted her injury might have been more extensive, but it was clear to me that God's Word was speeding up the healing process for me. Before I started therapy, I couldn't even reach up to get a glass from my kitchen cabinet, or raise my arm above my head to wash or comb my hair. I claimed God's promises and put action to my faith by daily applying the doctor's instructions. I used a pulley to raise my arm up and down.

I remember another therapist who almost always worked with her patient right next to the table where Brent worked on my shoulder. I called her "they shiny-haired girl." She was a very attractive girl with the shiniest hair I had ever seen. On occasion, she filled in for Brent and worked with my shoulder. She always listened to me so intently with an expression of either "*wow!*" or disbelief, I don't know which. However, I do know she was soaking up my testimony on healing from cancer by the stripes of Jesus, and she knew I was looking to this same Jesus for healing of my shoulder. She saw that He is not only able but also willing to heal. Her patient was the woman who had undergone two manipulations and whose shoulder was still frozen. I

106

was there for only a short time and never had to have the manipulation...*only Jesus!*

The same faith that had healed me of breast cancer was bringing restoration to my injured shoulder. It didn't happen automatically. I had to do something both naturally and spiritually to work with the Word. I had to do the exercises and I had to continue to speak the promises instead of what I felt. The Bible compares our tongue to the rudder of a ship. Just as the tiny rudder guides a large vessel through the water, the words we speak with our tongue will guide our lives. If it's healing we want, we need to speak healing. If we need deliverance, we speak deliverance. If we desire prosperity, we must speak prosperity. Don't wonder or hope that what God says is so; for those who walk according to His Word, all of God's promises are yes and amen!

Developing Faith

Keeping our words lined up with God's takes discipline. Faith is developed the same way a bodybuilder develops his muscles: through training. We have been given the measure of faith which has been dealt to every man (Romans 12:3), but it's up to us how we use that faith. A bodybuilder adds the desired weight to his bar, increasing the weight as his strength grows and develops. If he left the same amount of weight on the bar day after day, he would never develop more muscles.

We, too, must put the desired amount of Word seed in our heart and continue to water it and remove any weeds. The weeds are doubts, wrong thinking, and wrong believing that will choke the Word. If the enemy can choke the Word then he can kill our seed.

Friend, God's Word is truth! What He says He will do. You must grab hold of that truth no matter what you might be facing. You are an overcomer through Christ. It's time to uproot unbelief! Working in your yard I am sure you had a weed that needed to be removed at one time or another. Maybe it was a dandelion. I have never seen such long roots on such small weeds. These roots grow deep, and if you aren't careful when pulling them up, you will break the root right off. If you don't get the whole root, then all of your efforts are in vain. What you have to do is spend time digging around the root to loosen the surrounding soil. Little by little, you can finally grab hold and pull the whole thing out, root and all.

God's Word and His wonderful promises work the same way. The more time you spend preparing the "soil" of your heart, the more effectively the Word can work to bring the promised victory! Keep planting your faith, water it with your words, and watch it grow into a bountiful harvest. Don't grow weary in well doing: for in due season you shall reap, if you faint not! (Galatians 6:9).

Chapter 7

The Shadow of Death

Five months had passed and Charlie and I were still celebrating the Lord's victory in our lives. One never forgets to maintain a thankful heart after having been down such a challenging road.

We were busier than ever with our catering business, and had received a catering contract at one of the local Catholic schools where we prepared lunches for the children kindergarten through eighth grade every day. It was early February when the Holy Spirit began telling me, "Get back into the healing scriptures, you're going to need them."

I certainly saw no signs of a problem, but I knew the voice of the Holy Spirit and heeded His words. I started bringing a Walkman with me to the school where we prepared the lunches, and listened to Sister Copeland's healing scriptures every day. That's when it happened: I started having severe vaginal bleeding. Immediately, I phoned my

OBGYN's office. "That's a 'red flag' considering your history," they told me, and made an appointment for me the next afternoon. The date was Tuesday, April 8, 1997.

The morning of the doctor's appointment, Charlie and I were in the school kitchen. I was standing at the gas stove listening to Sister Gloria talk about "Paul's thorn in the flesh." The Scriptures tell us that Paul's thorn was not some sickness or ailment; rather it was "a messenger sent from Satan to buffet him." Paul was traveling wherever the Holy Spirit led him to go, telling everyone about the love of Christ. Everywhere he went people were being saved in droves.

Satan doesn't like it when we begin to share Jesus with people. He will do anything and everything he can to stop us, even if it means he has to kill us.

I was telling everyone I came in contact with about the goodness of the Lord. I remember right after I had the breast surgery, I would go to the grocery store and make opportunities to share Christ with anyone who would listen. If I needed a watermelon for a catering job, for instance, I would ask someone to pick it up for me, telling him or her that I had just had surgery. That immediately prompted a sympathetic heart. The person would always be very helpful and curious at the same time. "Oh, what kind of surgery did you have?" they would ask.

That was just the door of opportunity I was waiting for! As soon as it opened I walked right on through and began to tell them how

God had healed me based on His Word. Each person was amazed, but at the same time showed some suspicion and doubt. Some of the individuals I shared with were already Christians; others were not. Often the Christians would look at me as if I had that third eyeball in the middle of my forehead, so you can imagine how the non-Christians reacted. Yet, I could still see the expression on their faces; a glimmer of hope shone because of what God had done for someone else. Maybe they or someone they knew was sick: their mother, father, or co-worker, and they thought, *Will God do the same for them...for me?*

We must always be ready and willing to share the goodness of God and what we've learned with someone else. We don't know what someone's needs might be at that very moment. Believe God to orchestrate such divine encounters for you. He loves people and cares about each and every detail of their lives. What a privilege to have a part in communicating His love to someone else. The Scriptures tell us that to whom much is given, much will be required. That is the way I felt about God healing my body. I knew much had been given to me and it was my responsibility to teach others.

A Spirit of Infirmity

As I listened to Sister Gloria that morning, it was as if something...*someone* rushed up behind me. I could feel the chilling breeze on my neck. For a moment, fright overtook my emotions. I didn't think anyone else was there, Charlie had left the room, *but*

111

perhaps it was one of the children or the maintenance man who sometimes played jokes, I thought.

As I turned to see who or what was there, I saw a big, dark shadow as it passed over my shoulder and moved out onto the floor. It was just like in the movies. A black shadow-like cloud seemed to float past me and evaporate as it moved across the floor tiles.

When Charlie came back into the room, I told him what had happened. He and I immediately agreed that the dark presence had to have been either a spirit of infirmity or a spirit of death. We took our authority, binding the spirit in its operation and strategy against me. We pled the blood of Jesus and stood on God's Word that no weapon formed against me could prosper, and that with long life God would satisfy me and show me His salvation. The Word was such a comfort to me through this most unusual encounter.

My regular physician, Dr. Presley, was not in the office the afternoon of my appointment. Instead, I was scheduled with Dr. Channell, a physician who had recently joined the group practice. We made our introductions and then visited about the two procedures he would be performing that day. First, he would do an ultrasound, then he would take the biopsy.

"If on ultrasound the endometrial tissue is more than ten centimeters," he warned, "that would not be good." As the procedure began, Dr. Channell was focused intently on the ultrasound screen. "Hummm," he let out a peculiar sound.

"So how many centimeters is it?" I asked. I anticipated it would be maybe twelve or thirteen centimeters.

Much to my amazement, he said, "Twenty-nine."

"That doesn't sound good," I told him.

He nodded his head, confirming my concern. "Let me show you what I'm seeing," he explained, as he turned the monitor for me to view the screen. "Here is your uterus and here is what I'm seeing." It was a line about the width of a pencil mark and measuring about one and a half inches long. I saw it with my own eyes, and indeed it looked threatening, even to someone with an untrained medical eye.

Dr. Channell made some notes, and then I met him across the hall for the biopsy. It was relatively quick and painless. After the procedure was complete, Dr. Channell had a disturbed and saddened look on his face. He told me, "Once the stage of cancer is determined, we will talk about what type of treatment will be necessary and how many treatments will be required."

As I got up from the examination table, I looked him square in the eyes and told him, "Dr. Channell, you don't know me. God already healed me of breast cancer last year and He can certainly do it again." I continued to tell him how I never missed a day's work due to any diagnosis, and this one would be no different. I don't think he knew quite how to take my unusually bold reply. He looked at me, smiled, and politely left the room.

Come Boldly to the Throne

I was not about to take a lie from Satan and crumble under it. That is exactly what these symptoms and results were: lies that did not line up with the Word of God. Earlier that very day Satan had tried to frighten me with the spirit of infirmity or the spirit of death. Obviously, he had forgotten that I am not moved by what I see; I am only moved by what I know through faith in God's Word, which says I am healed by the stripes of Jesus. If we waiver from the Word, Satan has us right where he wants us. I knew what I was up against, and I knew right where to go to get help—directly to the throne room. Hebrews 4:16 says, "Let us therefore come boldly unto the throne of grace, that we may obtain mercy, and find grace to help in time of need."

The scripture doesn't tell us to come begging and pleading with God for our help, it says to come *boldly.* We can only come boldly when we know that what God promises He will also perform.

Covenant Promises

The following Friday, April 11, I had been given instructions from Dr. Channell's office to call for the results of the biopsy. When I phoned, the nurse told me they hadn't received the results yet, and that I should call again on Monday. That could have been a long weekend if I had spent too much time thinking on the "might be's" and "could be's" instead of what God's Word says. I continued about my business, and that Saturday was setting up a luncheon for the "Understanding God and His Covenants" class. It was hard to imagine I had been doing the same thing just a year earlier and under similar circumstances.

Right before the group sat down to eat lunch, their instructor, Beverly, asked me to share the doctor's report. I shared what the doctor had said and then, just as I had done the year before, I asked those who could agree for my healing to pray for me. If they couldn't pray for healing, then I preferred that they didn't pray at all. That is neither rude nor arrogant; it is knowing my covenant promises and expecting God to keep them.

A Confirming Word

On Sunday morning, Charlie and I had gone to church. I was standing at the Welcome Center where I met Gary, assistant to the head of the Vietnam Veteran's Ministry Group at Christ Church, and an artist who painted the picture of Christ bent over a straight chair with the American flag draped over Him. I had only met Gary once or twice before, and he only lived in Nashville briefly. I will never forget the expression on his face that morning. It was as if he was glowing. His smile stretched from ear to ear as he greeted me with a kind hello. After a few moments had gone by without any dialogue, I finally asked him, "Gary, you know, don't you?"

"Yes, Deborah, I do," he responded. "As I stood shaving this morning, the Lord told me that I was to come and tell you that He is the same today as He was yesterday, and He will do the same for you as He has done before."

That was a word spoken in due season and it confirmed what Charlie and I were already believing. Oh, how that word bolstered my faith!

A Glorious Presence

That Sunday, Charlie and I were assigned to sit on the platform for the reading of the Word. As we sang and worshipped the Lord, it was as if God and I were the only two in the entire building. It was glorious! As I praised Him, I began thanking Him for healing me again. The presence of the Holy Spirit was tremendous. My physical body literally felt weak under the weight of His glory, and I just knew I would be slain in the Spirit.

After the service, a friend came to me and told me what he had witnessed during the worship. "Sis, I saw the glory of the Lord all over you and said to myself, 'Look at Sis go!' "

My friend Linda met me in the hall as I was heading downstairs. Her husband, Bob, and Charlie were heading to the Ukraine together later in the week to teach at the St. James Bible College in Kiev. "Have you seen Charlie?" I asked her.

"He's meeting with Bob," she told me, "they should be along any minute."

I proceeded to tell Linda about how the Spirit had visited me during praise and worship that morning. Tears began to roll down her face as she told me, "Deborah, I saw it. The glory of the Lord was all around you."

Just then, Charlie and Bob met us in the hall and we proceeded to Bob's office where they all laid hands on me and prayed for my healing. We all agreed that Satan was only trying to make Charlie's trip to Kiev difficult. He wouldn't want to leave me on Thursday with this most recent report from the doctor. Together, we stood firm; I was healed by the stripes of Jesus.

On Monday, I phoned the doctor's office for my test results, and once again, they didn't have any. This time they told me it would be seven to nine days before they would have any results and that I should call back at that time.

Heaven Answers

Tuesday afternoon I was out on my screened porch talking to the Lord. I told Him, "Lord, I know that You know I am going to a healing service tonight at Christ Church. I know that You know what time it starts. Lord, I am telling everyone I come in contact with that You are my healer and their healer. The people who come tonight need to see the evidence of my healing. I don't need evidence—I've got Your Word and that is enough for me. I know Your Word is truth and that You cannot lie. But Lord, the doctor's office said that I wouldn't have any results for seven to nine more days. I am asking You to do something and to do it now! It's not going to look good for

You if You don't. No one will ever believe me again if You don't demonstrate Your healing power now."

You mean you talk to God like that?

I did and I do. He has given me His Word and He expects me to believe it and hold Him to it.

Two and a half hours after my little "conference" with the Lord, the phone rang. It was Dr. Channell. He began to stumble over his words. "Deborah, they um…the pathologist who read the biopsy could not find the cancer anywhere," he said with wonder and amazement in his voice.

I remember yelling in the receiver, "Praise God! We have been praying for healing!"

The doctor tried to explain what he really didn't understand. To me this was yet another testimony of the life-giving power in God's Word! I had gone to God boldly on the basis of His Word, and heaven answered right on time!

Sad to say, nothing really happened at the healing service that night. Charlie and I met Becky and Gill, two powerful prayer warriors when we arrived at the church. They had been standing in faith with us for healing. As we shared the report, they began to praise the Lord. Laughter and joy filled the room where we were standing. Then the four of us prayed and thanked God that He sent His Word and healed us, and delivered us from our destructions.

We then joined the meeting, where the leader and counselors were in prayer. I waited with great excitement to tell them what had happened. But when they finished praying and I shared our news with the leader, there was not much of a response. Nothing was mentioned during the service either. I was determined for the classmates and counselors to know of this victory, so after the meeting I made my way around the church and told everyone I could.

With our timely answer, Charlie's heart was light as he and Bob left for the Ukraine. He knew that God was faithful to His Word and His promises, and that the protection based on those promises would preserve me in all my ways, bearing me up, lest I dash my foot against a stone.

Yes, he could now proceed with the trip and be a tremendous help to Bob, who was the instructor. Charlie would be able to share our victories over the last year with the students at the school, as well as with a family we had lived with in 1991 while on a mission trip. The mother and family were non-Christians; however, the twelve-year-old daughter was a believer. I remember sitting on the bed in her grandparents' home and walking her through the plan of salvation. She informed me that she had already accepted Christ at an earlier time.

The mother had a dream that she had seen me before Charlie and Bob got to her home. The next day, Charlie arrived with pictures of me, and just as in her dream, she saw me. She was so excited and just couldn't believe it. This event showed her that the God we believed in was real. If Satan could have kept Charlie from going to Kiev due to another surgery, the woman never would have experienced God—a God in whom she had not believed.

His Mercy Endures Forever

Dr. Channell scheduled another appointment for me to come back in one month. He wanted to follow up with me and make sure that everything remained clear. I had also made a prayerful decision to have a hysterectomy and a bladder tack. When I went back for my appointment, the nurse did another ultrasound and could not find the line of cancer that the doctor had originally shown me. What she did find, however, was a tumor the size of a tennis ball on my right ovary. I remember on a previous visit that Dr. Staggs, a doctor in the same practice, had mentioned the tumor to me. His face was serious and he told me eventually it would need to come out. That was all that was said, until now.

Surgery for the hysterectomy and bladder tack was scheduled on June 9, at 7:30 A.M. Charlie and I made the familiar trip to Baptist Hospital early that morning. My Mother and Peggy also drove up to be with us. Dr. Presley stopped in to speak with Charlie and me before the surgery, and he asked me if we could pray before they came to take me to the holding area. "Of course!" was my answer. God was so faithful, giving me a doctor who requested that we pray!

Then, the nurse came and wheeled me away while Mother and Peggy stayed to be with Charlie. I'm quite sure they had as much fun that day as they had the year before when I went in for the breast cancer surgery. Yes, you can have a joyful time when you know that you know that you know God supplies all of your needs—including healing—according to His riches in glory!

After the hysterectomy, the urologist was scheduled to do the bladder tack, and then I would be on the road to recovery. However, Satan had other plans. When I got back to my room, I began to experience intense nausea. I tried to eat a popsicle and that only made things worse. Several people came by to visit and I remember wondering how much longer I could keep feeling that way.

After one of our children left, I told Charlie that I could not continue like this and we needed to pray and cast off this spirit of nausea. We went right to the same Word that had been so faithful to me during the last surgery. The Word says in Matthew 12:29 that I could enter the strongman's house, bind him up, and spoil his goods. That is exactly what Charlie and I did. We bound the spirit of sickness and commanded it to leave my body. I had God's Word built into my heart, but I still needed to act on that Word to experience its power.

After we finished praying, I needed to settle my spirit. I shut everyone and everything out and began to focus on Jesus my Healer. Charlie had packed my Walkman and an assortment of scripture tapes and worship music, so I put on my headset and began to listen to praise and worship. I kissed Charlie, turned over and fell asleep. I awoke a new woman; the nausea had left my body and I was once again "whole in Jesus' name." The Lord is good, and His mercy endures forever!

The Desires of Our Heart

The day after the surgery, the urologist came in and I asked him why Dr. Presley had cut me vertically instead of horizontally. He explained to me that Dr. Presley's reasoning was that he felt the tumor was cancerous and he didn't want to "spread it all over." However, they had tested the tumor every possible way and could find no cancer cells present anywhere.

Dr. Presley never mentioned the tumor on the ovary. This, too, was another "messenger" of Satan to buffet me. Satan never stops; he is constantly at work trying to kill, steal and destroy. This was yet another of his tricks. No one mentioned the tumor, so there was no prayer covering this area of my body. Consequently, the devil tried to win. He is always seeking whom he may devour, but I had not given him authority over my mind or body.

Remember playing the game "Mother May I" as children? We lined up and the leader, the Mother, stood in charge in front of the rest of the children. The Mother asked a question and the children had to say, "Mother May I?" If someone moved before saying, "Mother May I," he was punished and sent backward so many steps.

I was playing no game with Satan. He was not going to gain any ground over my mind or body. He was trying to move, but I had taken authority over him when speaking God's words in faith. God's words penetrated my body leaving no part uncovered, not even an ovary.

Following the surgery, I spent the next few weeks at home recovering. The time I spent with the Lord was precious. Some days I literally thanked and praised Him all day long. I sensed His presence ever so close to me. The Word is true: As we draw near to Him, He draws near to us (James 4:8). How I wish everyone could experience this intimate fellowship with the Father, Son, and Holy Spirit. It's available, and He longs for it. All it takes is time.

I know many people who believe that God makes us sick to "teach" us something. I certainly learned a lot when sickness attacked my body, but it had nothing to do with the sickness. I learned things because for the first time in my life I desperately searched God's Words for answers. I learned that Jesus is the Healer and God has nothing but good gifts to give. Sickness comes from the devil—the oppressor—whom Jesus defeated and gave us dominion over. The Holy Spirit could just have easily taught me these truths had I not been sick, if I had had ears to hear and eyes to see.

In my times of fellowship with the Lord during my recovery, He began to stir a desire in my heart to teach the truths I had learned about healing. I began to pray about teaching Healing Classes at Christ Church on Monday nights. I saw that there was a great need for people to learn what God's Word teaches about the healing power of God, not only physically, but emotionally and spiritually too.

To God's glory, the class became a reality! I had the privilege of seeing people healed, restored, delivered, and built up in their faith in

123

God's Word. As we delight ourselves in Him, He truly does give us the desires of our heart!

Chapter 8

Suffering in the Flesh

When I refer to "suffering in the flesh," I don't mean that we suffer through sickness. We suffer because we don't know what the Word of God says about the health and healing that belong to us. If we don't know that Jesus bore our sickness and carried our pain, how will we walk in this blessed promise?

If we are honest, the truth is most of us do not spend enough time in the Word to really know what God says concerning His healing promises. We don't plant God's Word in our heart, abide in it, and allow that Word to abide in us. We don't make the Word of God and our relationship with Him first place, and consequently, something other than the Word reigns in our life.

It is often a good idea to take a self-inventory to evaluate what the priorities are in our life. Who is in control of our life? Is it us, our circumstances, our family or friends? Or can we truly say that God is in control? The scriptures tell us that the Holy Spirit is to control our lives. Galatians 5:16–17 says, "This I say then, Walk in the Spirit, and ye shall not fulfill the lust of the flesh. For the flesh lusteth against the Spirit, and the Spirit against the flesh: and these are contrary the one to the other: so that ye cannot do the things that ye would."

Our flesh and the Holy Spirit within our born-again spirit are constantly at odds. What the flesh wants, the Spirit never wants, and what the Spirit desires, the flesh never agrees with. It's not easy to make the flesh obey what is right, but when we have been diagnosed with a sickness or disease we have to make a choice. Will we go to the Word and take the necessary time to find out what God says about healing, or will we let the enemy lie to us and tell us there is no hope?

The Bible says God's words are "life" and "health" or "medicine" to all our flesh. Whatever is put in our heart will eventually come out of our mouth and be produced in our life. If we are consumed with watching television and know every sit-com on prime-time, every item previewed on QVC or clip on Home & Garden because we have already seen them, what do you suppose we will be talking about? If most of our spare time is spent shopping, playing, or simply sitting around wasting time, God's medicine will not be working in our body. If we want to benefit from God's medicine, we have got to be faithful to take His medicine.

Choices, Choices, Choices

The words we speak significantly affect our life. In fact, I am convinced that our words can change our immune system. God said in Deuteronomy 30:19–20:

> **I call heaven and earth to record this day against you, that I have set before you life and death, blessing and cursing: therefore choose life, that both thou and thy seed may live:**
>
> **That thou mayest love the Lord thy God, and that thou mayest obey his voice, and that thou mayest cleave unto him: for he is thy life, and the length of thy days: that thou mayest dwell in the land which the Lord sware unto thy fathers, to Abraham, to Isaac, and to Jacob, to give them.**

We choose what comes out of our mouth, whether blessing or cursing, life or death. The Holy Spirit's role is to prompt us to make correct choices, but His job is not to force us to make them. The Holy Spirit is a gentleman. It is flesh or the devil that will try to force, control, or manipulate us. God created us with a free will, but unfortunately, we are self-centered people. We generally want what our flesh wants and it's always easier to go with the flesh. Such a choice, however, can be deadly.

Recall what Hosea 4:6 says: "My people are destroyed for lack of knowledge." And James 1:17 tells us that every good and perfect gift comes from above." Healing is a gift from God, but if we allow the enemy to keep us ignorant of what the Word says we have, then the devil has accomplished his goal and we have chosen a path of destruction.

Thank God, He gave us His Word in Psalm 107:20, which says, "He sent his word and healed them, and delivered them from their destructions."

God sent us His Word! He made provision for our healing and deliverance from the hand of the enemy. When we know the Word we can boldly say, "I shall not die, but live and declare the works of the Lord!" (Psalm 118:17)

I have seen words change situations either to better or to worse. For example, people who struggle with a poor self-image lack self-confidence and often think and speak the worst about themselves. People who have an image of themselves in poor health—even though they may be in perfect health—will speak as if they are in poor health. They speak negatively instead of positively and eventually their body responds accordingly.

We can generally pinpoint what someone believes based on what he or she says. If we ask, "How are you?" and a person responds by telling us how bad off he or she is, it's a fairly good indication that the person does not know the power of his or her words. Proverbs 18:21 says, "Death and life are in the power of the tongue: and they that love it shall eat the fruit thereof."

What we believe and speak not only affects our body, but also our immune system. Our words become either a blessing or a curse to us and are vital to our health and well-being.

The following verses give scriptural foundation for the connection between our health and the words that we speak.

> **Thou shalt also decree a thing, and it shall be established unto thee: and the light shall shine upon thy ways.**
>
> **Job 22:28**
>
> **The mouth of a righteous man is a well of life: but violence covereth the mouth of the wicked.**
>
> **Proverbs 10:11**
>
> **The words of the wicked are to lie in wait for blood: but the mouth of the upright shall deliver them.**
>
> **Proverbs 12:6**
>
> **A man shall be satisfied with good by the fruit of his mouth: and the recompence of a man's hands shall be rendered unto him.**
>
> **Proverbs 12:14**

There is that speaketh like the piercings of a sword: but the tongue of the wise is health.

Proverbs 12:18

He that keepeth his mouth keepeth his life: but he that openeth wide his lips shall have destruction.

Proverbs 13:3

In the mouth of the foolish is a rod of pride: but the lips of the wise shall preserve them.

Proverbs 14:3

The tongue of the wise useth knowledge aright: but the mouth of fools poureth out foolishness.

Proverbs 15:2

A wholesome tongue is a tree of life: but perverseness therein is a breach in the spirit.

Proverbs 15:4

A man's heart deviseth his way: but the Lord directeth his steps.

Proverbs 16:9

The heart of the wise teacheth his mouth, and addeth learning to his lips.

Proverbs 16:23

Pleasant words are as an honeycomb, sweet to the soul, and health to the bones.

Proverbs 16:24

I create the fruit of the lips; Peace, peace to him that is far off, and to him that is near, saith the Lord; and I will heal him.

Isaiah 57:19

For verily I say unto you, That whosoever shall say unto this mountain, Be thou removed, and be thou cast into the sea; and shall not doubt in his heart, but shall believe that those things which he saith shall come to pass; he shall have whatsoever he saith.

Mark 11:23

And the tongue is a fire, a world of iniquity: so is the tongue among our members, that it defileth the whole body, and setteth on fire the course of nature; and it is set on fire of hell.

James 3:6

These references are more than just words; they carry life-giving power! Second Timothy 3:16–17 says, "All scripture is given by inspiration of God, and is profitable for doctrine, for reproof, for

131

correction, for instruction in righteousness, that the man of God may be complete, thoroughly equipped for every good work."

Medical science aids healing through physical means by administering medicines or therapy. God's healing is administered through the human spirit. Notice First Corinthians 2:9–12:

> **But as it is written, Eye hath not seen, nor ear heard, neither have entered into the heart of man, the things which God hath prepared for them that love him.**

> **But God hath revealed them unto us by his Spirit: for the Spirit searcheth all things, yea, the deep things of God.**

> **For what man knoweth the things of a man, save the spirit of man which is in him? even so the things of God knoweth no man, but the Spirit of God.**

> **Now we have received, not the spirit of the world, but the spirit which is of God; that we might know the things that are freely given to us of God.**

It's our spirit that must receive the Word of God, and that comes by faith: what we believe in our heart and confess with our mouth. Faith comes by hearing and hearing the Word. Faith is the warranty deed, that thing for which we have fondly hoped is ours at last! Even when we don't see the results of what we believe, we believe God's Word is true because faith is the evidence of things "not seen."

Believe the Word

It's our choice to believe God's Word or not. But when we make a decision to pick sides against God's Word, we have no right to blame God and say His Word didn't work for us.

Do you remember being in PE class when you were younger? You lined up to be picked for the dodge ball or softball team, and the team captains literally chose the classmates they thought would be the best players for their team. These players were chosen because the captains believed they were the best, and of course, with the best players their team would have a better chance of winning the game.

In order for God's Word to work for us, we must make a decision to agree with it and to "choose" the yoke destroying power of God's Word in order to defeat our opponent. Mark 11:24 says, "Whatsoever things you desire when you pray, *believe* that ye receive them and you shall have them."

Jesus also said, "And all things whatsoever ye shall ask in prayer, *believing*, ye shall receive" (Matthew 21:22). Notice He didn't say, "...whatsoever ye shall ask in prayer, *hoping*...." We must make a quality decision to believe God and be determined to win the battle against the enemy.

Proverbs 4:20 admonishes us to pay attention to God's words and incline our ears to His sayings. If we don't take the time to pay attention to, listen to, and receive God's words in our heart, we will never experience their power in our body.

Before the captains of the dodge ball or softball teams chose the classmates to play on their teams, they first spent some time watching those classmates play. They saw the classmates' determination and listened to their excitement about the game. They heard them cheer and play with an expectancy of winning the game. Those were the classmates the captains chose. They never picked the ones who didn't have any pep in their step. They didn't pick the ones who were complaining about being out in the hot sun or who wished they didn't have to play. No, they picked the ones who were determined—expectantly believing, not hoping—to win the game. We must not pick sides against God and His Word. God's words are mighty and they "win" every time we make a decision to believe them.

Proverbs 4:20 goes on to say "do not let them (God's words) depart from thine eyes." In other words, read, read, read, study, study, study. Keep those words in your heart, because out of the abundance of your heart, your mouth will speak.

God's words are life to those who find them. "Find them" suggests that we have to diligently search for them. That means the words are not going to jump from our Bible and attach themselves to our body.

God's words are health to all our flesh. I heard an example about God's words being health or medicine to our flesh and it bears repeating. A woman was very sick so she went to the doctor. The doctor wrote her a prescription for some medicine with specific instructions for when and how many times each day she was to take the medicine. Time went by and the woman wasn't getting any better so she went back to the doctor. "Well, did you take the medicine as I instructed?" he asked her.

"No," she replied. "But I rubbed the bottle all over my chest three times a day."

Obviously that is not going to help the woman, just as healing is not going to work for us unless we take God's medicine as prescribed. The Word of God cannot be health to either soul or body before it is heard, attended to, and received. God's words are life to those who *find them.* If we want to receive life and healing from God, we have to take time to find the words of scripture that promise these results. We can't do that while watching television five hours a night, shopping at the mall, or talking on the phone two or three hours at a time.

Make a decision to be on God's team. Take the necessary time to be a "team player." Learn to use the time you have profitably. If you have a tape player in your car, listen to teaching tapes on your drive to and from work. Play praise and worship tapes, the Bible on tape, and healing scriptures on tape. Keep the Word going into your ears at every opportunity.

After I was diagnosed with breast cancer and gained a revelation of healing through God's Word, I began to pump the Word into my ears and heart from the time I woke up in the morning until the time I went to bed at night. I also did as Hebrews 4:16 says and came boldly before the throne of grace to obtain grace to help in time of need. I had a need and went boldly before the Father and told him I didn't want to die, I wanted to live.

God honors His Word! When we trust God's Word as we would natural medicine, and make a decision to apply the Word to our situation by faith, then we can see that His Word does exactly what it says it will do. I am living proof!

Abide in the Word

Healing is a very individual event. It's between you and God and no one else. We can't expect someone else to obtain healing for us. Jesus said in John 15:7, "If *ye* abide in me and my words abide in you, ye shall ask what ye will, and it shall be done unto you." When God's Word becomes engrafted in your spirit, it has become part of you and cannot be separated from you. The same way that a doctor takes skin from one part of a person's body and grafts it to another part where it then lives, the Word now lives in your flesh by the faith in your heart. God's Word concerning healing taking root in your flesh becomes greater than the disease. The result is health and healing for your body in the name of Jesus. The authority of God's Word will give you the confidence that not only is God *able*, but He is *willing* to heal you.

And this is the confidence that we have in
him, that, if we ask any thing according to
his will, he heareth us:

And if we know that he hear us, whatsoever we ask, we know that we have the petitions that we desired of him.

1 John 5:14–15

When we believe and speak God's Word from our heart, we are operating in faith. Hebrews 11:3 tells us the worlds were literally *framed* or *created* by the Word of God. Without words, God would not have created anything.

Our words create an image that we will eventually live out. Every time we speak the Word of God, that image becomes stronger and more powerful. When we are seeking healing, we speak the Word that has been engrafted in our heart and agree with it. John 6:63 says, "It is the Spirit who gives life, the flesh profits nothing. The words that I speak to you they are spirit and they are life."

Romans 8:11 says, "But the same Spirit of Him who raised Jesus from the dead dwells in you."

Satan is the author of sickness and disease. James 4:7 tells us to "submit ourselves to God, resist the devil and he will flee." Our job is to submit to God, not to television, to things or to our job. We are to glorify God in our body and our spirit, which are His. God told his people in the old covenant "So you shall serve the Lord your God and He will bless your bread and your water, and I will take sickness away from the midst of you."

How much more will He do in the new and better covenant?

Deborah M. West

Don't listen to Satan.

Don't side in with him by speaking negatively about the problem.

Stay in the Word!

Say what God says.

Believe you receive and you will have!

Chapter 9

How to Activate Your Faith

Now faith is the substance of things hoped for, the evidence of things not seen.

Hebrews 11:1

We have taken time to study the Word of God and to learn what the Word says about healing. Through precept and example, we have discovered that healing belongs to us. We have also learned that the Word tells us what we must do to receive this precious gift that Jesus purchased for us.

All of God's promises come only one way, and that is by faith. Hebrews 11:6 confirms, "But without faith it is impossible to please him...." When it comes to any of God's promises, faith is the hand that reaches out and receives what Jesus has obtained, the Holy Spirit has secured, and God the Father has so willingly provided.

139

Faith vs. Hope

How are we going to have faith? The Bible says we already have "the measure of faith" (Romans 12:3). This implies that our faith can grow. Faith can develop and gain strength just as a muscle does.

So how do we get more faith? As we have learned in Romans 10:17, "Faith comes by hearing and hearing the Word of God."

Some might ask, "How do we know we are truly in faith and not just *hoping* that what God promised He is able also to perform?"

Let me show you what the Word says. "Faith is the substance of things hoped for, the evidence of things not seen," as our opening text reads. Notice the verb "is" in this verse is used in the present tense. Hope is always future tense. So if we want to determine whether we are in hope or faith, it's simple. If it's not *now*, it's not faith! If we say, "I sure *hope* I will be healed," that's not faith, that's hope.

Perhaps we are hoping for finances to meet a particular need. Faith—the substance of things hoped for—gives us the assurance that we will have the money when we need it based on what the Word of God says in scriptures such as Philippians 4:19: "My God shall supply all your need according to his riches in glory by Christ Jesus."

If we need physical strength to do a certain job, faith says, "The Lord is the strength of my life."

Faith has a voice and it always says what God says. If God says it, it is so! If we want God's Word to work for us, we must agree with His Word because the Word always works and faith cannot fail.

Jesus told us in Mark 11:24, "What things soever ye desire, when ye pray, believe that ye receive them, and ye shall have them."

According to this verse, when do we receive? When we see what we have prayed for manifest? No, we believe we receive *when we pray*. Faith says, "Healing is mine, deliverance is mine, victory is mine...*now!*"

Believe the Word instead of siding in with the circumstances, and your faith *will* turn to sight. Circumstances change, feelings are fickle, but God's Word stands forever! "For ever, O Lord, thy word is settled in heaven" (Psalm 119:89).

Faith vs. Doubt

When we're walking through a healing, we can encounter many obstacles. I know you might receive a bad report, but if and when you do, say what the Word says instead of what the doctor's report says.

"But people will think I'm crazy!" some might argue.

What do you care what anyone thinks?

Faith-filled words change seemingly impossible circumstances as we saw in Mark 5. We read in an earlier chapter how Jairus, a ruler of the synagogue, appealed to Jesus to heal his daughter who lay at the point of death. Time was of the essence, but as Jesus started on his way to Jairus's house, a woman with an issue of blood reached out with the hand of faith, received her healing and delayed the Master.

No sooner had Jesus commended the woman, telling her, "Thy faith hath made thee whole," than some men came from Jairus's house with a bad report. "Your daughter is dead, why trouble the teacher any further?" (v. 35)

As soon as Jesus heard the word that was spoken, He said to the ruler of the synagogue, "Do not be afraid; only believe." (v. 36)

Imagine what Jairus was going through. In desperation he had pushed his way through the crowd to get to Jesus with his need. He fell at Jesus' feet, begging him to come and heal his little girl. He didn't care what the people thought; he had faith that would not be denied.

But then came the woman interrupting Jesus on the way to Jairus's house. I imagine Jairus was thinking, "I wish Jesus would leave her alone and come on!" The longer Jesus stood and talked to the woman, the more Jairus's faith had an opportunity to wane. But Jesus knew just what He was doing. I am quite sure He knew Jairus's struggle, and as soon as Jesus heard the doubters declare that Jairus's daughter was dead, He braced Jairus's faith: "Do not be afraid, only believe." Jesus knew that if Jairus believed their report and allowed words of doubt to escape his lips, his faith would weaken and dissipate.

Jesus permitted no one to follow Him to Jairus's house except Peter, James and John the brother of James. In other words, Jesus put the doubters out, both those on the way to Jairus's house as well as the weeping wailing bunch that filled the house. Then, Jesus brought the child's parents and the men in faith with Him in to her room. He reached down, took her by the hand, and said to her, "Little girl, I say to you arise." And she got up!

Now that is faith in action! Jesus knew that it was God's will for this little girl to live, and He knew that He had come to do His Father's will. Raising the little girl from the dead was a divine display of God's will revealed through Jesus, the Living Word.

Jairus was much like I was when I was diagnosed with breast cancer. The more I saturated myself with the Word, the more my faith grew to the point I didn't care what people thought. I pressed through obstacles of doubt in my path to make it to the Master. I knew what God's will was and is concerning healing, and I wanted to do everything possible to agree with His will and receive His words in my heart.

When you or someone you love and care about is in desperate need, you don't care what other people think. Jairus had heard about Jesus and the miracles He had performed, for the Bible says, "Jesus' fame went about the region." Jairus was doing just what I did. He had believed the words of the Word made flesh, received them, acted on them, and by them his daughter was raised from the dead!

Get yourself in a position to receive what God's Word says, then act on the Word by speaking it out of your mouth. Hold fast to the confession of your faith without wavering, for He who promised is faithful (Hebrews 10:23)!

Jesus' Healing Touch

Some years ago at Christ Church, we had our Wednesday night prayer meeting in the Wallace Chapel. At that time it was an intimate meeting of about two hundred people. We would come together to praise and worship the Lord, and to usher in the Holy Spirit.

One particular Wednesday night, Donnie Wood make an announcement that we would be having a healing service the following Wednesday. Charlie and I didn't know God's Word pertaining to healing at that time in our lives. We knew how to stand in faith for our material needs, but as far as knowing the scriptures and standing on them for physical healing, we had not a clue.

At that time I had not been diagnosed with cancer; however, I did have a need for healing of my lower back. When I was a teenager, I had been involved in a car accident with my former husband. After he and I married, I continued to suffer with back pain. The pain was so bad that at times I couldn't even get out of bed to use the restroom.

When Donnie announced the healing service, I got so excited. I told Charlie I wanted to shout at the top of my lungs, "Extra, extra, read all about it! Jesus is coming to Christ Church next Wednesday night for a healing service!" I could just see all the people lining up outside the doors—those with diseases, the crippled, and those in need of deliverance. I pictured it being just like when the Bible described Jesus' fame going out and all the people coming to Him to be healed.

"Charlie," I boldly declared, "next Wednesday night I am going to go down and receive healing of this lower back pain."

I just couldn't wait!

Wednesday night finally came. We were all in the chapel singing praises to the Lord. Wouldn't you know it, negative thoughts began to flood my mind. Satan is such a liar. He will stop at nothing to talk us out of what is ours. As I stood there singing, the devil told me, "Surely, you are not going to go down tonight. You did that just a few weeks ago and those same people are here tonight. They saw you go down then. They will think you're stupid for going back again."

The longer we sang the closer I came to accepting Satan's lies. I remember grasping the pew until my knuckles turned white and thinking, *I am not going to go down.* There was such a spiritual battle going on. Suddenly, I muttered just under my breath, "Satan, you let go of me. I am going down to accept this healing."

Charlie and I were sitting on the right side of the chapel, three rows back. I knew when I got up to go to the altar that Charlie wouldn't follow me. He is always right by my side, but he knew this was something I needed to do by myself. I stood up, walked across the front of the church to the other side, and knelt down to pray. As I offered up prayers of thanksgiving, I heard Donnie say to the people that if anyone wanted to pray at the altar to come. I had a sense that Charlie would come down to me at that time.

The pain became so great as I knelt there that I had to stand to get some relief. As I stood and worshipped the Lord, I knew without a

145

doubt that Jesus had come to deliver me from the pain. I could sense Charlie's presence somewhere behind me. Donnie was praying aloud and as his words filled the sanctuary, I felt heat across my lower back. I assumed someone had placed their hands on me and I was hoping it was Charlie, as the placement was halfway down my bottom.

After the service I asked Charlie, "Did you have your hands on my lower back?"

"No," he told me.

"You mean that wasn't you?" I said in disbelief.

"No, it wasn't me," Charlie insisted.

"Charlie, whoever it was had their hands almost on my bottom."

The following Sunday, I was leaving the chapel when I ran into a friend who had been at the Wednesday night healing service. "Barbara," I asked her, "you were standing behind me last Wednesday at the healing service; was that you who had your hands on me?"

"No, Deborah. It wasn't me and there was no one between you and me. I didn't even touch you."

At that moment I knew Jesus the Healer had touched me that night, just as He had touched *the every, the many, the multitudes,* and *the one.* I had made a decision a week before the healing service that Jesus would be there. Jesus doesn't come to pick and choose whom He will heal; He said He heals *all who will receive.* All I needed was a point of contact. When I said with my mouth that I knew Jesus would be there, I activated my faith and made a point of contact where I believed I would receive. By faith I knew that I knew He was going to perform His Word.

God is just waiting for us to get it together and stand firm on His Word. Make a decision today to get into the Word and receive what God has provided for you.

Speak God's Word

I pray that the power of God's Word is becoming more and more real to you. His Word contains the same resurrection power that raised Christ from the dead, translated us from death to life, and breathes quickening power into our mortal bodies!

God's words formed *you* and every bit of life on this planet. God created the whole world with words! He believed and He spoke the worlds into existence (Hebrews 11:3). We receive healing for our bodies the same way: by believing and speaking God's words.

Jesus knew the power of the words He spoke. Notice the following references.

1. "Arise little girl." Matthew 9:18–26
2. "Arise, take up thy bed and walk." Luke 5:17–25
3. And Jesus rebuked the demon out of him and healed him. Luke 8:26–39
4. "What do you want Me to do for you?" Mark 10:46–52
5. "Come forth Lazarus." John 11:1–44
6. "I am willing, be cleansed." Luke 5:12–13
7. "Stretch out your hand." Luke 6:6–10

8. "Woman, you are loosed from your infirmity." Luke 13:10–12

9. "Go show yourselves to the priest." Luke 17:11–14

10. "You deaf and dumb spirit, I command you, come out of him and enter him no more!" Mark 9:14–25

Speak God's Word! Don't *hope* you are going to be healed some day; *believe* you receive *when you pray*. Most of us have heard these words or said them ourselves: "I *hope* the doctor's report will be fine." Or "I *hope* I am able to walk to the door when I get there." Or "I *hope* I'll be able to take the medicine, the radiation, or the chemotherapy without them making me sick."

People, there is power in the words you speak! Don't *hope* the doctor's report will be fine; *believe* the report of the Lord! He came to heal the sick, raise the dead, and set the captives free! Don't *hope* you can take the medicine without getting sick. *Know* that with God *all things* are possible. There is a difference between hope and faith, and when you cross over, you know it!

I took twenty-five radiation treatments and seven radiation boosters. I prayed and quoted God's Word every day before I ever got to the hospital. I thanked God for my deliverance from any negative side effects. I refused to go home and be defeated by the enemy. I didn't have to be defeated because God's Word says that Jesus heals, if only we believe! Healing and victory are ours, purchased and won by Jesus the Son!

We can boldly confess that, "Surely he bore our sickness and carried our pains." There is power in the Word of God, power through the name of Jesus, and power in the blood that He shed for you and me. Jesus said in Matthew 21:21–22, "Assuredly, I say to you, if you have faith and do not doubt, you will not only do what was done to the fig tree, but also, if you say to this mountain, be removed and be cast into the sea, it will be done. And all things, whatever you ask in prayer, believing you will receive."

Jesus told us to say to the mountain, "Move," and it will move. I don't mean we just name and claim whatever we please, I mean we find out what God has provided and stand on His Word until that which we have believed has manifested. Be steadfast in God's Word. Satan works around the clock trying to make our lives a complete failure and he never takes a vacation. He knows if he can keep us out of the Word of God that we will always be defeated. So what does he do? He has us making cookies for the church bake sale, making food for the shut in, and attending every meeting the church has to offer. All these are good things, unless they are keeping us from learning and applying God's Word to our life.

Mountain-Moving Faith

We must develop mountain-moving faith! Joshua is a prime example of such faith in Joshua 3. Joshua and the children of Israel had come to the river Jordan and were lodging there before crossing over. After three days they were ready to cross over to the other side, but the river was at flood stage and there was no convenient way around it. Regardless of how deep the water, they had no choice but to cross the river. This is after they had been in the wilderness following the miraculous escape from Egypt. All of their needs had been met by God, but one more obstacle stood between them and the Promised Land. God could easily have caused the river to subside right before their eyes; He could have thrown up a bridge for them to cross. But He didn't do either of these things. Instead, He gave Joshua some strange orders to pass on to the camp.

1. Camp officers ordered the people to keep an eye on the ark of the covenant. As soon as they saw the priests carrying the ark they were to fall in behind it. (v. 3)

2. Joshua told the people to expect amazing things to happen. (v. 5)

3. Joshua commanded the priests to pick up the ark and stand in the river. (v. 6)

Giving such orders took faith on Joshua's part. Just as God has given us, He gave Joshua the instructions to fight the battle. God was very specific in telling Joshua what to do. Joshua didn't call his friends over to the river bank and tell them how terrible things were. He didn't cry "poor me, now what am I going to do?" He didn't sit around and talk about his problems. He received instructions from God and he obediently acted on them.

The Lord said He would provide dry ground for them to cross over, but these priests may never have seen a river this close before.

Remember they had been in the wilderness. Perhaps they couldn't even swim. They didn't remember seeing the Red Sea part; they hadn't been born yet. I imagine this river didn't look too friendly at flood stage. With all twelve tribes of Israel at their heels, it would be difficult for the priests to change their minds once they stepped in and the river kept flowing. In spite of all the problems, the priests acted on the word of the Lord given to Joshua and stepped in the river.

And as they that bare the ark were come unto Jordan, and the feet of the priests that bare the ark were dipped in the brim of the water, (for Jordan overfloweth all his banks all the time of harvest,)

That the waters which came down from above stood and rose up upon an heap very far from the city Adam, that is beside Zaretan: and those that came down toward the sea of the plain, even the salt sea, failed, and were cut off: and the people passed over right against Jericho.

And the priests that bare the ark of the covenant of the Lord stood firm on dry ground in the midst of Jordan, and all the Israelites passed over on dry ground, until all the people were passed clean over Jordan.

Joshua 3:15–17

God didn't give the priests absolute proof or overwhelming evidence that the waters would part. He did nothing until, by faith, they put their feet in the water as a step of commitment and obedience to the Word of the Lord. Only *after* the priests acted on the Word did God stop the flow of water. Mountain-moving faith will be given to us as we step out and follow the Lord's directions.

How do we pray a mountain-moving prayer? We get our eyes off the mountain and get our eyes on the Mountain Mover! Then, we step out in obedience on His Word that cannot fail. God told us we could move the mountains in our lives if only we would believe. As we walk with God, our faith will grow, our confidence in Him will increase, and our words will carry power to produce the desired result!

Numbers 13 tells us about the children of Israel perched on the edge of the Promised Land. They sent out twelve spies to survey the land, ten of which came back talking doom and gloom. "You wouldn't believe the size of the cities, the armies, and the giants! We had better look somewhere else," they said. However, two spies returned with a different report, saying, "The God who is faithful promised He would give us this land, so let's go in His strength and possess what belongs to us."

Ten looked at the size of the mountain; two looked at the Mountain Mover. Probably every person alive is standing in the shadow of a mountain that just won't move. Maybe the mountain is a destructive habit such as drugs, smoking, or drinking. Perhaps it's a character flaw, an impossible marriage or work situation, a financial problem, or a physical disability. Have you stood in the shadow of this mountain so long that you have grown accustomed to the darkness? Are your words filled with doubt and despair? God knows what your mountain is, and He doesn't need for you to tell Him again. He is waiting for you to return His Word to Him so He can perform it in your behalf (Isaiah 55:11).

Focus your attention on the Mountain Mover. His glory, power, and faithfulness will change that hopeless situation for you. Praise Him. Offer up praises of thanksgiving before you see the evidence. Start walking in faith, following God's leading, and watch the mountain be cast aside. The Word tells us, "Be anxious for nothing, but in everything by prayer and supplication, with thanksgiving, let your requests be made known to God; and the peace of God, which surpasses all understanding, will guard your hearts and minds through Christ Jesus" (Philippians 4:6).

When darkness seems to have fastened its grip, choking out the very light and life you have been believing for, be encouraged by the biblical account of Lazarus in John chapter 11.

> **Now a certain man was sick, named Lazarus, of Bethany, the town of Mary and her sister Martha.**

(It was that Mary which anointed the Lord with ointment, and wiped his feet with her hair, whose brother Lazarus was sick.)

Therefore his sisters sent unto him, saying, Lord, behold, he whom thou lovest is sick.

When Jesus heard that, he said, This sickness is not unto death, but for the glory of God, that the Son of God might be glorified thereby.

Now Jesus loved Martha, and her sister, and Lazarus.

When he had heard therefore that he was sick, he abode two days still in the same place where he was.

Then after that saith he to his disciples, Let us go into Judaea again.

His disciples say unto him, Master, the Jews of late sought to stone thee; and goest thou thither again?

Jesus answered, Are there not twelve hours in the day? If any man walk in the day, he stumbleth not, because he seeth the light of this world.

But if a man walk in the night, he stumbleth, because there is no light in him.

These things said he: and after that he saith unto them, Our friend Lazarus sleepeth; but I go, that I may awake him out of sleep.

Then said his disciples, Lord, if he sleep, he shall do well.

Howbeit Jesus spake of his death: but they thought that he had spoken of taking of rest in sleep.

Then said Jesus unto them plainly, Lazarus is dead.

And I am glad for your sakes that I was not there, to the intent ye may believe; nevertheless let us go unto him.

Then said Thomas, which is called Didymus, unto his fellowdisciples, Let us also go, that we may die with him.

Then when Jesus came, he found that he had lain in the grave four days already.

Now Bethany was nigh unto Jerusalem, about fifteen furlongs off:

And many of the Jews came to Martha and Mary, to comfort them concerning their brother.

Then Martha, as soon as she heard that Jesus was coming, went and met him: but Mary sat still in the house.

Then said Martha unto Jesus, Lord, if thou hadst been here, my brother had not died.

But I know, that even now, whatsoever thou wilt ask of God, God will give it thee.

Jesus saith unto her, Thy brother shall rise again.

Martha saith unto him, I know that he shall rise again in the resurrection at the last day.

Jesus said unto her, I am the resurrection, and the life: he that believeth in me, though he were dead, yet shall he live:

And whosoever liveth and believeth in me shall never die. Believest thou this?

She saith unto him, Yea, Lord: I believe that thou art the Christ, the Son of God, which should come into the world.

And when she had so said, she went her way, and called Mary her sister secretly, saying, The Master is come, and calleth for thee.

As soon as she heard that, she arose quickly, and came unto him.

Now Jesus was not yet come into the town, but was in that place where Martha met him.

The Jews then which were with her in the house, and comforted her, when they saw Mary, that she rose up hastily and went out, followed her, saying, She goeth unto the grave to weep there.

Then when Mary was come where Jesus was, and saw him, she fell down at his feet, saying unto him, Lord, if thou hadst been here, my brother had not died.

When Jesus therefore saw her weeping, and the Jews also weeping which came with her, he groaned in the spirit, and was troubled,

And said, Where have ye laid him? They said unto him, Lord, come and see.

Jesus wept.

Then said the Jews, Behold how he loved him!

And some of them said, Could not this man, which opened the eyes of the blind, have caused that even this man should not have died?

Jesus therefore again groaning in himself cometh to the grave. It was a cave, and a stone lay upon it.

Jesus said, Take ye away the stone. Martha, the sister of him that was dead, saith unto him, Lord, by this time he stinketh: for he hath been dead four days.

Jesus saith unto her, Said I not unto thee, that, if thou wouldest believe, thou shouldest see the glory of God?

Then they took away the stone from the place where the dead was laid. And Jesus lifted up his eyes, and said, Father, I thank thee that thou hast heard me.

And I knew that thou hearest me always: but because of the people which stand by I said it, that they may believe that thou hast sent me.

> And when he thus had spoken, he cried with a loud voice, Lazarus, come forth.
>
> And he that was dead came forth, bound hand and foot with graveclothes: and his face was bound about with a napkin. Jesus saith unto them, Loose him, and let him go.
>
> Then many of the Jews which came to Mary, and had seen the things which Jesus did, believed on him.

The moment Jesus said to the Father, "I thank thee that thou has heard me," the raising of Lazarus was complete in the spirit realm before it was seen in the physical realm. That's what we do while we are still contending with symptoms of sickness. God says that healing is already ours, and the healing process begins the moment we pray and believe we receive.

Sickness is not yours: don't claim it as your own!

Don't take possession of what belongs to Satan and what Jesus already took for you!

Possess the healing that has been purchased with the precious blood of Jesus Christ!

God's Will Revealed

Jesus sought not to do His own will, but the will of Him that sent Him (John 5:30). He said, "...he that hath seen me hath seen the

Father…" (John 14:9). Therefore, when Jesus healed the multitudes day after day, we saw the Father revealing His will. If healing is not for *everyone*, how can we pray the prayer of faith for *anyone?* If it is not God's will to heal all, then no man can be certain of God's will for himself. Since faith is expecting God to keep His promise, how can the sick have faith for healing if there is no promise in which they can confidently trust? The scriptures tell us how God heals the sick. "He sendeth His Word and healed them and delivered them from their destruction," Psalm 107:20.

We have already established that God is able to heal. But faith rests on more than mere ability. Let me give you an example. Suppose we were having a meeting and a millionaire came in and said to us, "I am able to give each of you $1 million dollars." This would not be a basis for us to have faith for the money, because faith does not rest on ability. If I were to ask each one of you if you were assured of getting the $1 million dollars, you might answer, "Well, I need the money and I hope I will be the lucky one, but I cannot be sure." However, if the millionaire says, "It is my will to give each of you $1 million dollars tonight, then we would all have grounds for faith to believe, and we would all say, "Thank you very much, I will take my money."

Now suppose God was a respecter of persons and that it was His will to heal only *some* needing healing. Notice in the following scriptures which of the sick ones Jesus healed.

And Jesus went about all Galilee, teaching in their synagogues, preaching the

gospel of the kingdom, and healing all kinds of sickness and all kinds of disease among the people.

Then His fame went throughout all Syria; and they brought to Him all sick people who were afflicted with various diseases and torments, and those who were demon-possessed, epileptics, and paralytics; and He healed them.

Matthew 4:23–24

When evening had come, they brought to Him many who were demon-possessed. And He cast out the spirits with a word, and healed all who were sick, that it might be fulfilled which was spoken by Isaiah the prophet, saying: "He Himself took our infirmities And bore our sicknesses."

Matthew 8:16–17

Then Jesus went about all the cities and villages, teaching in their synagogues, preaching the gospel of the kingdom, and healing every sickness and every disease among the people.

Matthew 9:35

And when Jesus went out He saw a great multitude; and He was moved with compassion for them, and healed their sick.

Matthew 14:14

And when the men of that place recognized Him, they sent out into all that surrounding region, brought to Him all who were sick, and begged Him that they might only touch the hem of His garment. And as many as touched it were made perfectly well.

Matthew 14:35–36

Then great multitudes came to Him, having with them the lame, blind, mute, maimed, and many others; and they laid them down at Jesus' feet, and He healed them.

So the multitude marveled when they saw the mute speaking, the maimed made whole, the lame walking, and the blind seeing; and they glorified the God of Israel.

Matthew 15:30–31

And great multitudes followed Him, and He healed them there.

Matthew 19:2

162

The "unlucky ones" were also brought to Jesus and received healing the same as the "lucky ones." Matthew tells why Jesus made no exceptions: "He healed them all, that it might be fulfilled which was spoken by Esaias, the prophet saying, 'Himself took our infirmities and bore our sicknesses.' "

Search the gospels for yourself and note the "ALL's" and "EVERY's." Healing was and still is for all. No one ever asked Jesus for healing in vain. Everyone who asked, received. Never was there a multitude large enough to have in it even one whom Jesus wanted to remain sick and would not heal. It was the multitudes coming for healing that caused the need for more laborers to be sent forth into His harvest to preach, teach, and heal. If this were not so, the twelve would have been sufficient.

When the disciples could not cast out the demons in the epileptic in Mark 9:14–29, we see that it was because of their unbelief. Peter, after having traveled with Jesus for three years, described Jesus' earthly ministry in this brief and profound statement: "…God anointed Jesus of Nazareth with the Holy Ghost and with power, who went about doing good, and healing all that were oppressed of the devil, for God was with Him" (Acts 10:38).

Healing Is Yours!

The Word shows us with infallible proof that it is God's will to heal *everyone, all the time*. Under the law, *all* included the Jewish people who met the conditions recorded in Exodus 23:25–26. "So you shall serve the Lord your God, and He will bless your bread and your water, and I will take sickness away from the midst of you. No one shall suffer miscarriage or be barren in your land; I will fulfill the number of your days."

For us under the new covenant, Jesus fulfilled the law, being made a curse for us according to Galatians 3:13, so that the blessing of Abraham now belongs to those who believe. In the new covenant, healing belongs to *all those who believe it and receive it!*

Faith for the healing of your body is the same as faith to believe for salvation. Faith for the healing of your body is the same as faith for believing that God forgives all your sins. Faith is the evidence of things not seen. You have not seen God wiping away your sins with a big eraser, but you know He said in His Word that your sins are forgiven.

If you are the beneficiary of a rich relative, you become wealthy the moment that person passes away, before you ever see the money. Everything in our Lord's last will and testament is already ours by virtue of the death of Jesus, the Testator. Faith is simply the way God designed for us to obtain what already belongs to us.

Healing is yours!

Meditate on that truth. Apply God's Word to your situation and watch it change your circumstances. Base everything on the promises of God and not on what you hear, see, or feel. If you think healing has passed away, it probably has for you because you don't believe.

It is impossible to please God without faith. Don't let your emotions keep you from walking the road of faith to your promised victory. The Word will train your flesh, if you will get into the Word and begin to apply it to your life. Walk the Word and your life will never be the same again!

About the Author

After being miraculously healed of cervical, breast and uterine cancer strictly by attending to God's

Word, Deborah West was commissioned by God to share her powerful testimony of healing, restoration and hope with those suffering from sickness and disease.

Raised up by the living Word of God, Deborah is passionate about her purpose. As president and co-founder of Deborah West Ministries, she boldly teaches how to remain steadfast and immoveable in the face of any circumstance by trusting in the living Word of God.

A preacher and teacher of God's Word, and author of her first book, *By His Stripes,* Deborah is committed to proclaiming the faith message through conferences, workshops, Bible studies, teaching tapes and the printed page.

Deborah and her husband, Charlie, enjoy a blessed home and church life in historic Nashville, Tennessee.

Deborah West asks that you contact Deborah West Ministries in Nashville, Tennessee for additional information regarding the following :

1. For Speaking engagements

2. for printed materials and a guide to product resources by Deborah West

        Deborah West Ministries

        P.O. Box 1925

        Brentwood, Tennessee 37024

Phone: (615) 332- WORD

Fax :   (615) 833-0555

Email: dwestministries@bellsouth.net

Web page: www.dwestministries.com

Printed in the United States
R381300001B/R3813PG16778X00002B/2